NASM CPT Study Guide!

Certified Personal Trainer Exam Prep Practice Questions for the National Academy of Sports Medicine

By Jenny Schaefer

Introduction	4
Basic and Applied Sciences and Nutritional Concepts	18
Assessment	36
Program Design	49
Exercise Techniques and Training Instruction	68
Professional Development and Responsibility	89
Client Relations and Behavioral Coaching	99
Randomized Practice Questions & Answers	149

Chapter 1

Introduction

In today's world, where the need to stay healthy and fit is unrepentantly increasing, the need for a personal trainer is also growing in the same vein. More people are now becoming aware of the significant role that a well-trained personal trainer can have in ascertaining one's fitness and health. However, another problem suffices.

Finding the right trainer has been a significant concern for lots of clients. There are people out there who have one knowledge or two about the nitty-gritty of being a personal trainer. Unfortunately, they deliver way below the expectation of the clients.

Go online. Do a quick survey. You would find so many tales of unpleasant experiences that many people have had with poorly trained personal trainers. To avoid more of these experiences, people are now more critical about the qualification of personal trainers before they hire them at all. One of the best ways to verify such qualifications is by certification.

Certification goes a long way in the authenticity of something or someone. In this case, a good certification from a reputable institution such as the NASM can go a long way in proving that you are experienced and knowledgeable enough to produce great results as a personal trainer. So, if you are interested in doing well as a personal trainer, a NASM certification will do you well.

About the NASM

As a fitness training provider, the NASM has its headquarters located in Gilbert, Arizona. Originally founded by Robert M. Goldman in 1987, the NASM operates as a subsidiary of Ascend Learning. Micheal Clark, who joined NASM as a partner in 2000, currently serves as the NASM CEO. He is the physical therapist for the NBA club, Phoenix Suns.

The NASM is widely known by many as the world's leading resource in the health and fitness industry. For over three decades, the institution has devoted itself to providing high-quality programs to certify personal trainers worldwide. Today, NASM certification is one of the most desired by employers in the personal trainer industry.

The significant certification offered is the CPT, which stands for Certified Personal Trainer. This certification can be affixed to a personal trainer's name as proof that such a trainer has undergone the necessary training under the NASM and is now a certified personal trainer.

Becoming a NASM-CPT is an excellent step towards becoming one of the top personal trainers out there. Apart from that, it also opens you up to numerous opportunities as you would now be viewed as a competent member of the personal trainer industry. However, to get this certification, you must take the NASM-CPT certification exam.

National Commission for Certifying Agencies (NCCA) is fully accredited to the NASM Certified Personal Trainer (NASM-CPT) certification exam. It also has the accreditation of the Institute for Credentialing Excellence. Besides, the NASM is registered with the Better Business Bureau as a sole proprietorship. This gives it all the backing it needs to stand out as one of the best certifications you can get in the industry.

Luckily, you can become a NASM-CPT in just a few weeks. The industry continues to grow as more and more people are now opting for a healthier lifestyle. Your chances of securing high-paying jobs and great opportunities are improved as a NASM-CPT.

Becoming a NASM certified personal trainer is one of the best decisions you can make as a professional. I'd tell you that one for free. Candidates who successfully pass the exams and can obtain the necessary credentials are permitted to use the certification credential "NASM-CPT" behind their name.

They are also allowed to use the title **"NASM Certified Personal Trainer"** whenever and wherever it is required. You can display your titles on office signage, resumes, websites, and business cards. You can also include it in your presentations, introductions, and even electronic signatures. However, the use of your NASM credentials should always be within the context of demonstrating professional credibility and not for endorsements or personal purposes.

Having the NASM CPT title gives you an extra edge amidst the multitude. For over 30 years, NASM has remained a hub for some of the best-quality personal trainers in the world. It has also become well-known for the scientific rigour of its certification exam program. Successful candidates can attest that the NASM program can help you improve your training expertise.

Over the last decade, almost 200,000 personal trainers have undergone the NASM training program and have received certification. Due to the model of the NASM program, it can train almost anyone eligible to take the exam. The NASM program is based on an exclusive Optimum Performance Training (OPT™) model. This makes it possible for candidates to encounter *"an industry-first comprehensive training system based on scientific, evidence-based research."*

Sure, becoming certified with the NASM will help you maximize your skills and improve your ability to help your clients achieve great results beyond ordinary expectations. Let's not forget to mention the innumerable career opportunities it avails you. A sure-fire step to becoming one of the best, most respected, and highest-paid personal trainers in the industry is to become a NASM Certified Personal Trainer.

Getting Familiar with the NASM Certification Program

When it comes to certification for education, solutions, and tools for health and robustness, the NASM has set the standard for sports performance and sports medicine professionals. The organization has pioneered first-of-its-kind solutions that are based on health and fitness for improving physical wellness.

NASM can serve thousands of people worldwide and positively impact the lives of a lot of people. Through continuous development and psychometric review, the NASM can provide the highest quality certification program. This program is an industry-accepted process that ascertains one's competency and proven effectiveness in the field. The NASM program is handled by top professionals in the area, including practitioners, educators, and psychometricians.

The NASM certifications are recognized as the industry's standard. This is why it is highly sought after by both clients and personal trainers alike. To become certified, you need to have a working knowledge of human movement science and functional anatomy. It would help if you also understood physiology and kinesiology. Candidates would be required to be abreast of functional assessment and the program design.

The NASM also offers certifications in advanced specializations fields. Some of them include the Performance Enhancement Specialist (PES) and Corrective Exercise Specialist (CES). Besides, more than 20 other education courses are offered by the NASM in various disciplines. They also provide education partnerships as well as professional fitness consultation services. There are also programs for practitioners at different levels of expertise, either beginner or advanced.

The program is directed at personal trainers who perform individualized assessments and design safe, effective, and individualized exercise and suitable conditioning programs. The NASM CPT program is prepared to design exercise and conditioning programs scientifically valid and based on clinical evidence. They help clients become better in terms of personal health, wellness, and physical performance goals. I need to highlight that personal trainers do not diagnose or treat areas of pain or disease. On the contrary, they will always refer clients with such needs to health care professionals.

Eligibility Requirements

Although almost anyone can understand the NASM CPT program, it cannot be taken by everyone. Candidates must meet specific eligibility criteria before they can be qualified to take the certification exam and receive the certificate. Here are some of the eligibility NASM CPT criteria:

- Before a candidate can receive certification, he/she must have a high school diploma or must be within 90 days of completing it. Other equivalents such as the General Education Development test (GED) or any other accepted test within the state are also accepted.

- Applicant must have obtained and maintained the Adult CPR as well as AED certifications. Applicants would also provide evidence of current CPR/AED certification before they can take the NASM exam. A current CPR/AED card will be required from already certified professionals applying for recertification.

Some of the approved providers include the American Heart Association, American Red Cross, American Safety and Health Institute.

- The only time a candidate can complete the certification program without fulfilling the certification requirements is if such a candidate requests an exception to eligibility requirements to sit for the certification exam. This can be only be done when an Exception Request/Appeal form is tendered along with other supporting documents.

This request will be looked into by the NASM Disciplinary & Appeals Committee. This is a committee of the Certification Governing Board. The Committee's decision, delivered in writing, may be submitted to the NASM Certification Governing Board for reconsideration. However, this might take a while because the board only meets three times annually.

- While the NASM does not require candidates to be 18 years of age before sitting for the certification examination, most clients often request liability insurance before employing a personal trainer. However, this insurance cannot be obtained by someone below 18 years of age.

Only NASM certifications make use of the above requirements. Hence, they must not be confused with any eligibility to practice requirements set forth under state law, regulation, or the rule of law or regulation of any other government or oversight body.

Taking the Exam

The whole process begins with commencing the initial enrollment. Due to the NASM CPT's extensive requirements, only 180 days from the initial enrolment is allowed for the preparation. Candidates will be given 180 days to obtain their CPR/AED certification and all other requirements.

However, if a candidate cannot make it due to specific situations, such a candidate can apply for a Program Extension by contacting NASM Member Services.

Once you are ready enough to take the certification exam, you must register for an exam date. Do note that the NASM recommends that examination candidates register for their exam at least sixty (60) days before the anticipated examination date to allow adequate preparation time. The NASM CPT certification exam is conducted and moderated by PSI, an 3rd party independent testing company.

Vendor. After registration, await the confirmation of the examination location, date, and time directly from the test administration site. The proof will be required on the exam date, so you need to keep it close.

Applicants are advised to register for an examination date in advance. However, it should be no later than three days before your preferred date. This is because the availability of space at your preferred location and preferred date is subject to demand. If you would be writing the exams as an international candidate, you must allow 4-6 weeks to schedule.

What you need to get admitted into the examination

There are a couple of things you should note before going to the exam location. Without all of these in place, you might be allowed to take the exam. Some of these instances include:

1) When you are not registered to examine a particular date and time at a location.

2) When NASM cannot confirm your identity with a current and valid government-issued photo ID.

3) When you cannot present a current CPR/AED certification card.

You can take the exam at the exact date and location you indicated upon your registration, for starters. The NASM would not allow you to take the exam at a different time or place.

Also, you might not be admitted into the exam without presenting a current and valid government-issued photo identification as well as your exam date confirmation provided by the test administrator. The examiner will permit only the individual named on the exam registration roster to take the certification examination.

Finally, candidates must present a copy of a current CPR/AED certification card from an approved provider.

Getting prepared

In a bid to adequately prepare candidates for the examination, the NASM allows candidates to that a one-time trial of the CPT for free. They also provide them with online self-study learning tools. Online self-study is an essential learning tool. Candidates should grasp the program and what to expect from a personal trainer after taking the free trial.

What You Need to Know About the Scoring

To pass the NASM exam, you need to pass the cut score. This is the minimum score required to pass an examination. The criterion-referenced cut scores are set to establish minimum levels of competency for the NASM-CPT examination. Panels of subject matter establish these cut scores by experts who evaluate whether a minimally qualified candidate would correctly respond to each item on the examination, rating those items accordingly.

The NASM employs a pilot scoring period when an updated exam is released. The test result is released during the pilot scoring period. However, before this is released, there is a brief delay in the release scores or pass/fail results. This gives ample time for reassessment, allowing NASM's psychometricians to ensure candidates have scored appropriately. Once this has been completed, the NASM would then provide a full release of the test results, and candidates receive their marks upon the initial score.

Upon the completion of the web-based testing, the scoring commences immediately. While at the test center, the tested applicants would receive a result. This result would reveal to them whether they have passed or not. However, the scores will not be made official until the NASM correctly verifies them. They would also ensure that any form of an exam-related incident is reviewed. This is majorly done within approximately two weeks after the exam date.

Before the official release of the results, candidates can use this preliminary report to provide evidence to employers of a passing score.

The NASM adopts a scaled score method. The scaled scores can range from 0 to 100, as it represents a conversion of the candidate's raw score to compare different forms of the same examination. Using this method, the NASM can remain consistent in reporting passing standards by accounting for the examination form's difficulty level. The same level of performance is required to meet the scaled passing score of 70 regardless of which form of the exam a candidate takes.

Candidates taking the NASM CPT exams must have a scaled score of 70 or higher to pass the examinations covered here. For each exam, candidates will be required to attempt 20 pretest questions correctly. These are not part of the scored ones as they are solely used for future examinations as part of the continuous exam development process at NASM as required by NASM's accreditor.

The NASM doesn't give candidates who pass the exams their actual scores. They only provide candidates who fail the exam with their actual score as well as a breakdown. This would be instrumental when preparing for the retest.

The NASM CPT Job Guarantee

To help hit the ground as quickly as possible, the NASM offers a Job Guarantee to candidates who have purchased and completed any CPT programs. However, this guarantee is only afforded to the participants who fulfil specific outlined criteria.

- You must pass my NASM CPT Certification exam with a score of 70% or higher
- You must apply to at least three employers of personal trainers within 50 miles of my primary residence.

- You must complete and submit the Job Guarantee Request form within 90 days of completing my NASM CPT Certification Exam.
- If you qualify, NASM will refund you only the amount that you paid for the Job Guarantee.

FAQs

Question:

What is the number of questions on the CPT exam? What is the duration of the exam?

Answer:

There are 120 test questions in the exam. However, 20 of them are research-based questions. Luckily, they do not add to the total score of the result. The exam would last for 2 hours, and it has a scaled score of 70% pass mark or above.

Question:

Are there any special accommodations provided by the NASM for the remote exam?

Answer:

In compliance with the American Disabilities Act, the NASM offers reasonable accommodation for candidates that fit the disabilities requirement.

Question:

Does the CPT exam have an expiration date?

Answer:

Yes, it does. The registration expires 180 days after registration.

Question:

Is there a CPT practice exam?

Answer:

Yes. Dependent on which package was purchased, you may have one or more practice exams available to you for the duration of your enrollment period. You can locate the practise exam via your NASM Student Portal.

Question:

What are the required documents candidates need to have for the test?

Answer:

You would be required to show a valid, current government-issued photo ID, as well as a proper Cardiopulmonary Resuscitation (CPR) and Automated External Defibrillator (AED) certification*. The proctor will verify both credentials before you are permitted to begin the exam. Inability to provide these would result in a compulsory rescheduling of your exam.

Question:

What CPR/AED providers does NASM accept?

Answer:

NASM recommends the following organizations: American Heart Association, American Red Cross, American Safety and Health Institute,

St. John Ambulance, Emergency Care & Safety Institute, or Emergency Medical Technician.

Question:

Is an online CPR/ AED course accepted?

Answer:

No, hands-on assessment is required. However, hybrid courses are accepted.

Question:

When should I arrive for my examination?

Answer:

Candidates ought to arrive at the scheduled time. However, if a candidate is unable to start after 15 minutes, it would be marked as a no-show. A new time slot might be allocated.

Question:

Will I receive my exam score?

Answer:

Although your score won't be released unless you fail, you might get a score report after the test.

Question:

Can anyone see my exam score?

Answer:

No, NASM does not release exam scores.

Question:

I failed my exam. Can I purchase a retest? And when can I reschedule?

Answer:

You would have to purchase a retest for another examination.

Question:

When do I receive my certificate?

Answer:

An official certification would be sent between 4 to 6 weeks after the NASM CPT exam's successful attempt. However, candidates can access a digital certification after one business day.

Chapter 2

Basic and Applied Sciences and Nutritional Concepts

By now, you must be well familiar with the nuances of the NASM CPT exam. We should state that all that we treated in the first chapter was merely introductory. In this chapter and the successive ones, we would be going more into the actual content of the NASM certified personal trainer exam. You would also be exposed to many practice questions to stay on top of your game.

Preparation is essential when it comes to these sorts of tests. You need to have the proper knowledge, but you also need to be familiar with the modalities and questioning style. These factors determine whether or not you would have a successful attempt at the NASM CPT test.

The test is divided into six different content domains for easy breakdown. They include;

- **Basic and Applied Sciences & Nutritional Concepts (17%)**
- **Assessment (18%)**
- **Program Design (21%)**
- **Exercise Technique and Training Instruction (22%)**
- **Professional Development and Responsibility (10%)**
- **Client Relation and Behavioural Coaching (12%)**

The percentage score in front is the total representation of each section in the overall scoring. By this, we can see that the **Exercise Technique and Training Instruction** section takes a considerable chunk of the entire scoring. Next to it is the **program design, assessment,** and down to the bottom three.

For this chapter, we would be talking about the **Basic and Applied Sciences and Nutritional Concepts.** This aspect of the test assesses the candidate's knowledge of human anatomy, the role of exercise physiology with bioenergetics, exercise metabolism, and the various body systems (nervous, muscular, skeletal, endocrine, cardiorespiratory, digestive systems).

This domain tests a candidate's knowledge of the science and theory of nutrition and human biology. However, we feel NASM could have gone more in-depth with the coaching methodology around food and less on just the theory side.

Anyways, it would be best if you were concerned about what you find during the test. Pay attention to nutrition concepts like macro, micronutrients, and supplements.

The other half concerns human biology. The focus being human biochemistry, including energetics, metabolism, endocrine system, cardiorespiratory system. It also bothers about human biomechanics such as neurotransmission, kinesiology, and basic principles of biophysics.

This content area also includes biomechanics, the science of human movement, and motor development principles. It also involves macronutrients, micronutrients, hydration, caloric intake, and expenditure guidelines.

Energy measurement units, dietary recommendations, and various diets are also considered. NASM would also test the candidate on label reading, factors that may affect weight management physiology, and the uses, effects, benefits, and risks of popular nutritional supplements.

Nervous System

The body movement of the human system involves the coming together of the nervous, skeletal, and muscular systems. The nervous system feeds the body with sensory information called afferent and motor information, also known as efferent. The functional unit of the human nervous system is called the neuron. The nervous system can be primarily broken down into the CNS, which involves the brain and spinal cord, and the PNS, which involves the somatic and the autonomic.

The PNS, fully known as the Peripheral Nervous System, contains various kinds of sensory receptors. Some of these receptors include photoreceptios, nocicepthaveechanoreceptors, and chemoreceptors. The two primary sensory receptors include the muscle spindle and the Golgi tendon organ. Also, the Peripheral Nervous System can be easily divided into two major areas, namely the autonomic nervous system and the somatic nervous system. To function correctly, the NS needs various electrolytes such as potassium, magnesium, water, and sodium.

There are three different stages that motor skill development often occurs. They are called the cognitive development, autonomous development, and the associative development. Our human nervous system can experience more development as we grow from being a child into becoming an adult.

The Skeletal System of the Human Body

Not only does it provide support for the body, it is also essential in the protection of the internal organs. The skeletal system is majorly classified into two parts, namely axial and appendicular.

Our bones as humans are known to function as attachment sites and levers - rigid rods - which in turn helps us to move as the muscles contract.

Bone growth occurs throughout life and remodels itself with specialized cells called osteoblasts and osteoclasts. There are five categories of bones: long, short, flat, irregular, and sesamoid. The vertebral column has five distinct regions: cervical, thoracic, lumbar, sacrum, and coccyx. In between each vertebra is an intervertebral disc that acts as a shock absorber and assists with movement.

When one bone articulates with another and is categorized by its shape, structure, and function, joints form. The Osteokinematic describes the bone movement, and arthrokinematic describes the action at the joint surface. Synovial joints are unique with a synovial capsule and contain other connective tissues, such as ligaments and fascia, that provide support. Synovial joints have six classifications: gliding (plane), condyloid, hinge, saddle, pivot, and ball-and-socket joints. Exercise and proper nutrition can have a significant positive impact on bone mass in aging adults.

Muscular System

The muscular system links the nervous and skeletal systems and generates force to move the human body. Muscles have a complex structure that includes different layers of connective tissue that surround the contractile muscle fibers. Myofibrils consist of repeating sarcomeres as well as the myofilaments actin and myosin. These create muscle contraction called the sliding filament theory. Adenosine triphosphate is also needed to generate energy for this process.

Excitation-contraction coupling describes the steps in the muscle contraction process involving the nervous and muscular systems. The electrolyte calcium and neurotransmitter acetylcholine are engaged in the excitation-contraction coupling process. The all-or-nothing principle describes how a motor unit either maximally contracts or does not contract at all. Muscles involved with fine motor skills have motor units with fewer innervated fibers. Motor units engaged in gross motor control have motor units with more innervated fibers.

Type I: Slow-twitch muscle fibers are smaller in size, produce less force, and are fatigue resistant.
Type II: Fast-twitch muscle fibers are more extensive, produce more force, and fatigue quickly.

The Cardiorespiratory, Endocrine, and Digestive Systems

The cardiorespiratory system comprises the heart, blood, blood vessels, and lungs. The respiratory system includes the respiratory airways, lungs, and respiratory muscles. The heart is contained in an area referred to as the mediastinum. A regular heart rate ranges from 60 to 100 beats per minute. Each side of the heart has two chambers: **an atrium and a ventricle.**
The body will increase the heart rate in response to exercise and decrease the heart rate during sleep. The heart's electrical conduction system is responsible for its function and begins with the sinoatrial node in the right atrium. The

sinoatrial node is the heart's pacemaker and sends the electrical signal to the atrioventricular node and ultimately into the ventricles. The right atrium gathers deoxygenated blood returning to the heart from the body and then sends it to the right ventricle and lungs.

Oxygenated blood is sent to the left atrium from the lungs. In turn, it sends it to the left ventricle pumped into the body. Special valves are present in the heart to ensure that blood pumps in a one-way fashion. The pulmonary artery transports deoxygenated blood from the right ventricles to the lungs, whereas the pulmonary vein transports oxygenated blood from the lungs to the left atrium.

The carbon dioxide from the deoxygenated blood pumped into the lungs from the right ventricle is expelled to the environment through regular expiration as part of the normal integrated functioning of the cardiorespiratory system. The amount of blood pumped out of the heart with each contraction is called a "Stroke volume". End-diastolic volume is the volume of blood in the ventricle before contraction, whereas end-systolic volume is the amount of blood present in the ventricle after contraction.

Stroke volume is ultimately a product of end-systolic volume minus end-diastolic volume. Cardiac output is the volume of blood pumped out of the heart in a minute and is a function of both heart rate and stroke volume. Normal blood pressure is a systolic less than 120 mm Hg with a diastolic of less than 80 mm Hg. Arteries transport blood away from the heart to the body. In contrast, veins transport blood back to the heart, and capillaries function as an exchange channel between the vessels and bodily tissues.

Breathing (ventilation) is divided into two phases, referred to as inspiration and expiration. The respiratory system is tasked with bringing in oxygen, filtering air from inspiration, and subsequently oxygenating blood from the heart and exhaling carbon dioxide. A standard respiratory rate is 12 to 16 breaths per minute and relies on the primary respiratory muscles (diaphragm and intercostals). During regular inspiration, active contraction of respiratory muscles occurs, whereas relaxation occurs during expiration. During forced or heavy breathing, expiratory ventilation relies on secondary muscles to compress the thoracic cavity and move air out.

Diffusion is a term used to describe the process of getting oxygen from the environment to the body's tissues. Abnormal breathing patterns will affect exercise performance and may be identified by shallow breaths, which often are associated with the use of secondary respiratory muscles (sternocleidomastoid, upper trapezius, or scalenes). A respiratory rate of fewer than eight breaths per minute would be considered too slow (bradypnea), whereas a rate of greater than 24 breaths per minute is considered too high (tachypnea). The endocrine system is composed of glands that secrete hormones.

When hormones are released into the bloodstream, they are protected by transporters, which carry them to the intended organ or structure, where they bind with a receptor to stimulate a particular function. The hypothalamus and pituitary gland control a majority of tasks for the endocrine system. Cortisol, facilitated by the adrenal cortex, may aid in recovery from exercise and as a marker of overtraining.

Insulin and glucagon both function to control blood glucose levels and work opposite each other; glucagon aids in glucose metabolism, and insulin aids in the cellular uptake and storage of glucose. The catecholamines, which consist of epinephrine and norepinephrine, are immediately stimulated from the adrenal medulla in response to exercise.

Cortisol, considered a catabolic hormone, is produced by the adrenal cortex and is sensitive to blood sugar and sleep. Although testosterone levels decline with age, intensive exercise can stimulate them. Growth hormones are responsible for growth and development and lipolysis and are produced from the pituitary gland. One of the most potent of the anabolic hormones is the insulin-like growth factor, in which the liver responds to growth hormones binding on liver receptors.

Testosterone, growth hormones, and insulin-like growth factors are stimulated in response to anaerobic resistance training and vigorous aerobic activity (e.g., high-intensity training styles). Thyroid hormones serve numerous functions in the body, including metabolism and increasing bone mineral density through calcitonin secretion. Adequate sleep is a requirement for glucose metabolism, hormone function, and muscle recovery.

The digestive system consists of the oral cavity (head and mouth), the upper GI system (stomach, small intestine [duodenum, jejunum, and ileum], and the lower GI tract (large intestine, rectum, and anus), as well as the liver, gallbladder, and pancreas.

Ingested foods and liquids are first processed in the oral cavity, where mastication (the mechanical process of chewing and breaking down food) begins the digestive process. Once the food is broken down, it passes through the esophagus into the stomach, where gastric juices aid in digestion, kill bacteria, and turn food into chyme, which is then passed into the small intestine.

The small intestine has a crucial function of absorption of carbohydrates, lipids, calcium, amino acids, and iron. Additionally, electrolytes, including water, are absorbed into the small intestines. The large intestine absorbs electrolytes and vitamins and serves to pass waste from non-digested food into the rectum. While fluids are absorbed into both the small and large intestine, the large intestine uses water to help pass waste into the rectum. The liver, gallbladder, and pancreas produce and store digestive juices secreted into the small intestine to aid digestion. Evidence suggests that exercise can improve digestive function by increasing the transit time of food from the upper to the lower GI tracts.

Human Movement Science

Movement is described in three dimensions based on planes, including the sagittal, frontal, and transverse planes. Osteokinematic describes the observable movement, whereas arthrokinematic describes the action taking place at the joint itself.

Movement is described using biomechanical terminology that is universal to all professions in the allied health industry. The sagittal plane is an imaginary line that bisects the body into the right and left sides. Movements in the sagittal plane include flexion and extension and plantar flexion and dorsiflexion of the foot and ankle. The frontal plane bisects the body to create front and back halves. Movements in the frontal plane include:
- Lateral flexion of the spine.
- Eversion and inversion at the foot and ankle complex.

The transverse plane bisects the body to create upper and lower halves. Movements in the transverse plane include internal rotation and external rotation for the limbs, right and left rotation for the head and trunk, horizontal abduction and horizontal adduction of the limbs, and radioulnar pronation and supination.

Motions of the scapulae include scapular retraction, scapular protraction, scapular depression, and scapular elevation. Muscle actions are described as isotonic, isometric, and isokinetic.

We can break down isotonic muscle actions into concentric and eccentric phases. Also, our muscles can play the role of agonist, synergist, stabilizer, or antagonist, depending on the movement being performed. Closed-chain movements anchor the body to the ground or immovable object, whereas open-chain movement involves the distal limb moving freely in space. Placing a muscle in a shortened position or lengthening a muscle beyond optimal length may reduce force output. Optimal length is the position with a maximal overlap of actin and myosin filaments.

The stretch-shortening cycle involves three phases: the eccentric phase, amortization phase, and concentric phase. The term force-couple is used to describe muscles that work in a synergistic function around a joint. The local muscular system involves muscles that generally attach on or near the spine and provide stability for the LPHC. The global muscle system can be broken down into subsystems, including the deep longitudinal, posterior oblique, anterior oblique, and lateral subsystems.

The subsystems describe the integrated function of muscle groups to transfer force for complex multi-joint movements and stabilize the HMS. The amount of force produced by the HMS relies on muscle recruitment and the lever type of the moving joint. Lever systems are classified as first, second, and third class. Third-class levers are the most predominant levers in the human body. Muscle synergies describe the cooperative function of multiple muscles recruited by the nervous system to complete a given movement pattern.

Proprioception is the intrinsic awareness of movement and body position in space. Feedback can come from internal or external sources and aids the process of motor learning. Motor learning integrates motor control processes with practice and experience, leading to a relatively permanent change in producing skilled Movements.

Exercise Metabolism and Bioenergetics

The human body needs a constant supply of energy to function correctly and meet the demands of exercise. The energy molecule used to do cellular work is called adenosine triphosphate (ATP), and it is made from food substrates consumed in the diet. The first law of thermodynamics states that energy can neither be created nor destroyed, only converted from one form into another.

The fuels used to create ATP are glucose from carbohydrates, free fatty acids from fat, amino acids from protein, and ketone bodies. These fuels are mainly obtained through dieting. Carbohydrates in the diet are broken down into glucose, which can produce ATP quickly via glycolysis. Glucose is stored in glycogen; the amount of glycogen that the body can store is much less than the amount of fat that it can store. Free fatty acids are the by-products of the breakdown of stored or consumed fats. They are oxidized exclusively via the aerobic pathway, which uses oxygen to create ATP.

Amino acids are the by-product of protein breakdown or digestion. The body can metabolize amino acids via oxidative phosphorylation, but this is not typical in healthy people because protein is usually reserved for muscle building rather than ATP production. The liver produces ketone bodies during periods of low energy intake or low carbohydrate availability. They can be oxidized via the oxidative phosphorylation pathway to create ATP.

Exercise is categorized by two factors: **intensity and duration**. The higher the intensity of the activity, the shorter the duration must be. The body needs fuel to perform an exercise. This fuel comes from broken down through chemical reactions to provide energy (ATP) and heat. The ATP-PC pathway is the simplest and fastest way to generate ATP. This system can only support short-duration activities because the supply of PCs is limited. Glycolysis is an anaerobic process and generates ATP quickly, but not a tremendous amount. The end products of glycolysis are ATP and pyruvate, which can become lactate under anaerobic conditions.

Oxidative phosphorylation is a process that uses oxygen to create ATP from substrate

molecules at a relatively slow rate. Oxidative phosphorylation can use pyruvate (starting from glucose), fatty acids, amino acids, or ketone bodies as substrate molecules. This oxidative metabolism produces
carbon dioxide as a by-product, which is then exhaled. The most critical factors determining the type of energy use during exercise are intensity and duration.

The intensity and duration of activity are inversely related, which means that the duration must go down as intensity goes up. Steady-state exercise is defined as a situation in which a person engages in the same activity level, without increases or decreases in intensity, for several minutes. Intermittent exercise is defined as frequent changes in the work requirement (intensity) during an activity. Exercise increases metabolic rate and breathing rate increases in proportion to it.

When the breathing rate becomes too rapid to allow talking, the body has shifted to oxidizing almost exclusively carbohydrate to fuel the activity.
Lower-intensity activities use a higher percentage of fat as fuel but generally do not burn many calories unless performed for a very long time. Higher-intensity activities have a higher percentage of energy coming from carbohydrates and usually burn more total calories in a given time. Daily food (energy) intake needs to be adequate to maintain a healthy body weight, allow for proper bodily function, and support physical activity.

If daily food intake is matched to energy needs, a person is said to balance energy. Calories are the basic unit of energy provided by food, and the total number of calories that a person burns in a day is called the total daily energy expenditure (TDEE). The resting metabolic rate (RMR) is the minimum number of calories needed at rest to keep a person alive and meet all body's functional needs.

The thermic effect of food (TEF) is the number of calories used to digest a meal. Non-exercise activity thermogenesis (NEAT) involves burning calories in activities that are not structured exercises. Exercise activity thermogenesis (EAT) is the calories burned during structured physical activity or purposeful exercise.

Nutrition

Registered and licensed dietitians and nutritionists are authorized to provide nutrition counseling, medical nutrition therapy, and meal plans. Fitness professionals (who are not registered or licensed dietitians or nutritionists) can provide general nutrition guidelines, direct clients to credible nutrition resources, refer clients to dietitians and nutritionists, and provide accountability and support with dietary changes.

Credible and reliable nutrition information includes peer-reviewed research and scholarly sources. Protein is made up of 20 amino acids; 9 are essential and must be obtained via the diet. The role of protein is the synthesis of tissues, organs, hormones, enzymes, and peptides. Dietary sources of complete proteins include soy and animal foods, such as meat, poultry, seafood, and dairy. Plant-based, incomplete protein foods include legumes, grains, and vegetables. Protein contains four calories per gram.

The RDA for protein is 0.8 g/kg bodyweight (considered a minimum to maintain nitrogen balance). The AMDR for protein is 10% to 35% of total calories. Carbohydrates include simple sugars, complex carbohydrates, glycogen, and fiber. Carbohydrates are an essential energy source for exercising individuals and athletes. Dietary carbohydrate sources include plant foods and dairy, including grains, vegetables, legumes, fruit, milk, and yogurt. Simple sugars include monosaccharides (glucose, fructose, galactose) and disaccharides (lactose, sucrose, maltose).

Complex carbohydrates are long chains of glucose units called polysaccharides, which slowly digest and raise blood glucose levels. Sources of complex carbohydrates include starches, legumes, and vegetables. The glycemic index reflects the effect of a carbohydrate on blood sugar levels; low GI foods cause smaller rises in blood glucose compared to high GI foods. Glycemic load is a better indicator of a carbohydrate's effect on blood sugar levels because it accounts for the glycemic index and the number of carbohydrates consumed.

Carbohydrates contain four calories per gram. Glycogen is the storage form of carbohydrates in animals and humans. It is stored in the liver and skeletal muscle. Fiber is indigestible carbohydrates associated with various health benefits and includes both soluble and insoluble fiber. The AMDR for carbohydrates is 45% to 65% of calories in the diet. Fiber recommendations: 25–28 g of fiber a day for women (aged 19–50 years) and 30–34 g of fiber a day for men aged 19–50.

Lipids are commonly referred to as fats and include triglycerides, phospholipids, and sterols. Saturated fat sources include animal fats, full-fat dairy, coconut, and palm oil. Polyunsaturated fat sources include omega-6, which can be found in nuts, seeds, oils) and omega-3, found in fatty fish, flaxseed, walnuts, chia seeds, fortified milk, eggs, dairy from grass-fed cows, and green vegetables.

Monounsaturated fat sources include olives, olive oil, avocado, peanuts, and canola. Phospholipid sources include meats, egg yolks, seafood, poultry, soybeans, and grains. Sterols sources include cholesterol from animal foods, egg yolks, and plant sterols. Lipids contain nine calories per gram. The AMDR for lipids is 20% to 35% of total calories. Vitamins and minerals are inorganic compounds essential to regulating metabolic processes, such as energy metabolism. Deficiencies and insufficiencies can contribute to health issues. Vitamins include two groups: fat-soluble and water-soluble. Vitamins A, D, E, and K are fat-soluble.

Water-soluble vitamins include vitamin C and B vitamins (thiamin, riboflavin, niacin, folate, B12, pantothenic acid, biotin). A balanced diet with a wide variety of minimally processed foods will likely supply adequate vitamins. Minerals include significant minerals and trace minerals. Hydration guidelines for athletes include 12–16 oz of fluid every 10–15 minutes for activities longer than 60 minutes. Athletes should replace fluid at 1.25 times the amount of body weight lost during an event.

Sports drinks may be hypotonic (lower concentration than body fluids), isotonic (similar concentration as body fluids), or hypertonic (higher concentration than body fluids). Sports drinks are likely unnecessary for short-duration exercise lasting less than 60 minutes (unless in hot or humid temperatures). Strategy combinations help clients achieve their weight goals, primarily including modification of energy intake and physical activity. The first law of thermodynamics states that energy cannot be created or destroyed but only converted from one form to another.

Weight gain results from energy intake exceeds energy output, whereas weight loss results from energy output exceeding energy intake. Other factors that influence weight include sleep, medications, and endocrine disorders. Food labels convey information on products' nutritional value and content via the nutrition facts panel and the ingredients list. Food labels can help clients make informed decisions about how a food item contributes to their nutrition and fitness goals.

Fat loss requires a net calorie deficit to minimize mass and reduce TDEE due to adaptive thermogenesis. Adequate caloric intake, especially adequate protein intake combined with resistance training, remains an essential element for increasing muscle mass. Nutrition strategies for improved sports performance are numerous and include ensuring sufficient energy (calories) and macronutrient intake. Meal timing and hydration are also essential to maximize sports performance.

Supplementation

Dietary supplements are products (other than tobacco) intended to supplement the diet that bears or contains one or more of the following dietary ingredients: vitamins; minerals; herbs or other botanicals; amino acids; dietary supplements used by humans to supplement the diet by increasing the total dietary intake; or concentrates, metabolites, constituents, extracts, or combination of any previously described ingredient.

In the United States, dietary supplements are regulated by the FDA according to the Dietary Supplement Health and Education Act. However, supplements do not require review or approval before being marketed and sold. The fitness professional should understand the necessary components of the dietary supplement label, including the active ingredients, other ingredients, pertinent warnings, total contents, usage instructions, and serving size. You may use dietary supplements for health and performance goals. Dietary supplements explicitly used for performance are classified as ergogenic aids.

Individuals may use Vitamin and mineral supplements to correct or supply insufficient dietary intake to consume the DV each day. Vitamin and mineral intake should not exceed the UL unless by the direction of a dietitian or physician. Dietary supplements and other ergogenic aids may produce adverse effects or serious adverse effects. Such effects may arise from the dietary supplements themselves or a change to or the contamination of the products. Protein supplements are convenient methods to increase total daily protein intake, the most crucial consideration for protein intake. Protein needs depend on the activity level, body size, and body composition goal of the individual.

An effective dose of creatine is at least 0.03 g per kg body weight, but a typical dose of 5g per day ensures complete muscle saturation. An effective dose of caffeine is 3 to 6 mg/kg (1.4–2.7 mg/lb) per day. Banned substances may not always be illegal substances, and athletes must check with their governing body (such as the NCAA or WADA) before consuming a dietary supplement. It is also wise for athletes to choose a supplement with third-party verification from Informed Choice or NSF. It is beyond the scope of practice for a fitness professional to prescribe dietary supplements to clients to treat a medical condition or disease. It is appropriate for the fitness professional to provide general education about supplements or direct a client to consult with a dietitian or medical professional.

PRACTICE QUESTIONS

- **When would a trainer be permitted to offer counsel to a client legally?**

A. A personal trainer should always offer to counsel to his or her clients
B. A personal trainer should always direct his or her clients to a professionally licensed counselor
C. The client refuses to show any sign of development
D. If the client is always struggling to meet up with the scheduled training appointments

Answer:
The Correct Answer is 'B'. A personal trainer should always direct his or her clients to a professionally licensed counselor.

As a personal trainer, you must understand that your scope of practice is encapsulated in pre-exercise risk assessment, program design, fitness testing, instructions, as well as the goal(s) evaluation. Therefore, a personal trainer is not licensed to perform any role outside the auspices of these functions. As a personal trainer, it is not in any way your duty to diagnose or treat any client with any form of mental or physical conditions. Hence, at the sight of such cases, you would do well to refer such clients to the appropriate practitioners. You are liable to any issues that might occur if you take it upon yourself to engage your clients beyond the scope of your practice.

2. Of the following, which of the options is not a method of creating a proprioceptively enriched environment?
A. performing active isolation exercises
B. using a foam pad
C. balancing on one leg
D. exercising in the sand
Answer:
The Correct Answer is 'A'. Performing active isolation exercises.

All the other options 'B', 'C', and 'D' are all forms of exercises that are done with a proprioceptively enriched or unstable environment. This forms the core components of their training method. However, the active isolation exercises are solely designed stretches for the improvement of the ROM.

3. Of the following, which option is not a division of the spinal column?
A. Sternum
B. Sacrum
C. Coccyx
D. Thoracic
Answer:
The Correct Answer is 'A'. Sternum

The remaining options 'B', 'C', and 'D' can all be classified as segments of the spinal column. However, the sternum, on the other hand, is located at the anterior side of the ribcage.

4. Of the following options, which of them best describe the sliding filament theory?
A. A process whereby the electrical impulses slide from the CNS down the Jaxon of the neuron in order to initiate the contraction of muscles.
B. Thin and thick filaments that exist within the sarcomere move past each other; as a result, it produces shortened muscle and force production
C. A process of neural stimulation that causes a contraction of muscles
D. Troponin providing binding sites along the actin filament for both tropomyosin and calcium in a case where the muscles need to contract
Answer:

The Correct Answer is 'B.'. Thin and thick filaments that exist within the sarcomere move past each other, producing shortened muscle and force production.

The sliding filament theory bothers around the process of muscle contraction. This involves the shortening and production of force caused by the sliding of the myosin (the thin filament) and the actin (the thick filament). Other options 'A', 'C', and 'D' are primarily just neurological binding and action principles.

5. There are two hormones responsible for fight or flight in the human system. What are they?
A. growth hormone and testosterone
B. epinephrine and testosterone
C. epinephrine and norepinephrine
D. testosterone and estrogen
Answer:
The Correct Answer is 'C'. epinephrine and norepinephrine.

These two hormones are responsible for activating the sympathetic nervous system. Usually active in an emergency or stressful situations, they can increase the heartbeat rate and limit the activities of non-essential organs.

Other options are responsible for different things in the body. For example, estrogen and testosterone are responsible the sexual desire in both females and males respectively. Also, the growth hormones can also be considered as an anabolic compound that functions hand-in-hand with testosterone.

6. Proprioception makes use of the information from which of the following to provide information regarding the body position and movement?
A. chemoreceptors
B. sensorimotor integration
C. muscle synergies
D. mechanoreceptors
Answer:
The Correct Answer is 'D'. mechanoreceptors

Identification of positions and movements by the sensory units is a key area of proprioception. However, a chemoreceptor can only function well in the detection of chemical as well as molecular presence in the environments of the body. This is achieved via olfaction; a process that involves the sense of taste and smell. Muscle synergies refer to muscles that belong to complementary groups.

7. Which of these can be referred to as a sesamoid bone?
A. patella
B. humerus
C. vertebrae
D. carpals of the hand
Answer:
The Correct Answer is 'A'. Patella.

The patella or kneecap is a sesamoid bone because it is embedded within a tendon and acts as a protective structure. Other options 'B', 'C', and 'D' lack any of the qualities that are associated with the sesamoid bones.

8. Of the following options, which two factors can be said to make up cardiac output?
A. heart rate x systolic blood pressure
B. heart rate/stroke volume
C. heart rate x stroke volume
D. systolic blood pressure / diastolic blood pressure
Answer:
The Correct Answer is 'C'. heart rate x stroke volume

Cardiac output is the amount of blood pumped per minute, and a minute is the amount of time in which the frequency of beats or pumps is determined as the heart rate and the amount of blood therein determined as stroke volume. That means cardiac output is a product of the heart rate and stroke volume.

9. Which of the following is the fastest energy system?
A. ATP-PC system
B. Glycolysis
C. oxidative system
D. the Krebs cycle
Answer:
The Correct Answer is 'A'. ATP-PC system

This system activates as the first energy system when the body is engaged in work. It is an anaerobic system which is why it can get to work almost immediately in the absence of oxygen. It is the least complex of the energy systems, which further leads to it being the fastest. The Krebs Cycle, D, is not one of the 3 main energy systems, but rather a subsystem of the oxidative system, C, the most complex and thus slowest of the 3 main energy systems.

10. A fracture that is proximal to the head of the humerus is located where?
A. It is located at the top of the humerus
B. It is located on the left side of the humerus
C. It is located at the midline of the humerus
D. It is located at the bottom of the humerus
Answer:
The Correct Answer is 'C'. It is located at the top of the humerus

Proximal refers to the middle or center point, however, the head of the humerus is located at the top of the bone. So although proximal refers to a central location, the head is at the top of the bone.

Chapter 3

Assessment

This aspect examines the candidate's ability to pick and carry out the appropriate assessments and then record and interpret these results to develop an appropriate fitness program. These questions include static postural assessments, strength assessments, movement assessments, speed and agility assessments, physiological assessments, cardiorespiratory assessments, and body composition assessments. This content domain also appraises the candidate's knowledge of PAR-Q assessment, essential elements of medical histories, lifestyle questionnaires, medical risk factors, assessments of special populations, re-assessment criteria, and signs indicating a client needs a referral the condition being out of scope.

Knowing your client's position, abilities, and needs to achieve their goals are the topics and concepts Assessment handles. Assessment is a vital first step in addressing a client; thus, it is considered an important domain and treated accordingly. This field covers a wide range of assessment protocols and procedures for the PAR-Q and other questionnaire formats and more practical approaches such as the numerous strength tests (postural assessment, overhead squat, pull, push, etc.)

To ace this domain, you will have to study and understand the various assessment type, perhaps even give them a try in the real world so you can verify what the book claims with the skills you are actually equipping.

Health, Wellness, and Fitness Assessments

The general purposes of conducting physiological assessments are to collect baseline data to help fitness professionals develop personalized exercise programs. The PAR-Q+ is considered an appropriate minimal screening tool for conducting an HRA. Fitness professionals should also gather additional information through an HHQ that may prove helpful in selecting fitness assessments, designing exercise programs, and monitoring progress.

An HHQ includes information about a client's medical history (e.g., injuries, surgeries, medications, and chronic disease) and lifestyle habits (e.g., exercise, diet, sleep, stress, and occupation). Exercising and resting heart rate and blood pressure responses provide valuable information on health risks and training adaptations. Many anatomical locations can be used to measure a client's RHR. However, for accuracy, safety, and ease of administering, NASM recommends that
fitness professionals measure a client's radial pulse.

Blood pressure (BP) is elucidated as the outward pressure exerted by blood on the arterial walls. BP scores are important because higher scores indicate greater risks for developing cardiovascular disease, which can become life-threatening. The BP of an average person is lower than 120/80 mm Hg. Anthropometry is the field of study of the measurement of living humans for purposes of understanding physical variation in size, weight, and proportion. Many different anthropometric measures exist, including body fat assessments, BMI, and circumference measurements. Anthropometric measurements provide useful information related to predicting a client's risk for mortality and morbidity. There are many methods for measuring a client's body fat percentage, including underwater weighing, skinfold measurements, and bioelectrical impedance analysis.

While all methods are valid, bioelectrical impedance is arguably the most popular method used in fitness facilities for ease of use. Cardiorespiratory assessments help the fitness professional identify safe and effective starting exercise intensities as well as appropriate modes of cardiorespiratory exercise for clients. Examples of cardiorespiratory assessments include O2max testing, the YMCA 3-minute step test, the Rockport walk test, and the 1.5-mile run test. O2max testing is considered the gold standard for identifying a client's level of cardiorespiratory fitness, but it requires specialized equipment and training to conduct.

In addition, it requires the client to exert maximal effort. Consequently, this test is not
commonly used outside of exercise laboratories or medical facilities. The talk test is an informal cardiorespiratory assessment used to gauge the intensity of cardiorespiratory activity based on the client's ability to hold a conversation. The VT1 test is an incremental test performed on any device (e.g., treadmill, bike) that gradually progresses in intensity level and relies on the interpretation of how a person talks to determine a specific event at which the body's metabolism undergoes a
significant change. A key point to this protocol is to remember an aerobic test that aims to estimate the intensity where the body uses a balance of fuels (i.e., 50% fat, 50% carbohydrates).

The VT2 talk test measures the intensity where the body can work at its highest sustainable steady-state intensity for more than a few minutes.

Posture, Movement, and Performance Assessments

Static posture is typically assessed in a standing position and is used to identify the three postural distortions: pes planus distortion syndrome, upper crossed syndrome, and lower crossed syndrome. Pes planus distortion syndrome is characterized by flat feet, knee valgus, and internally rotated and adducted hips.

The lower crossed syndrome is distinguished by an anterior pelvic tilt and excessive lordosis
of the lumbar spine. Upper crossed syndrome is shown by a forward head and protracted shoulders. The OHSA is the first movement assessment performed for clients and serves as the
basis for all other movement assessments. It evaluates dynamic posture, core stability, and neuromuscular control of the whole body during a squatting motion. During the OHSA, notate all movement impairments to identify potential muscle imbalances. From the anterior view, look for feet turning out or knees caving in. From the lateral view, look for low-back arching, excessive forward lean of the torso, or arms falling forward.

The single-leg squat assessment should be used by clients who have performed well in the OHSA or if the fitness professional is considering single-leg exercises in their programming. This test is a good assessment of an individual's ability to balance, which is an essential functional consideration for daily living and exercise programming activities. Pushing and pulling assessments evaluate the function of the upper extremity and concurrent core stability. They can be used as an intake assessment or an integrated part of the actual programming. When performing pushing or pulling assessments, look for the following movement impairments: *low-back arching, shoulders elevating, or head jutting forward.*

Performance assessments can be requested by clients looking to measure maximal strength and improve athletic performance, power, muscular endurance, speed, and agility. Muscular endurance of the upper extremities can be measured using the push-up test during a pushing movement. The bench press and squat strength assessments measure maximal strength capabilities. These tests are advanced assessments for strength-specific goals and may not be suitable for clients with limited experience with resistance training. The vertical jump and long jump assessments measure lower-body power.

The LEFT test is designed to test lateral speed and agility. LEFT is considered an advanced assessment for speed and performance-specific goals. The 40-yard dash assessment evaluates reaction capabilities, acceleration, and maximal sprinting speed.

The pro shuttle (5-10-5) test assesses acceleration, deceleration, agility, and control. This test is most appropriate for clients with athletic goals seeking to assess agility and sprinting speed. All assessments need to be sequenced in a specific order to help guarantee accurate results. Non-fatiguing assessments, such as a preparticipation health screening and physiological and body composition assessments, should be conducted before posture, movement, cardio, and performance assessments. Fitness professionals should always use caution when implementing movement and performance assessments with their clients. Certain populations, such as overweight or obese, youths, older adults, and prenatal clients, may need to modify or avoid particular movement and performance assessments. Some assessments are not applicable because they do not relate to the client's goals. Other assessments may cause safety concerns.

Take it from me; if you are not assessing, you are making guesses. Assessments help personal trainers gather valuable information about their clients. The information gathered includes objective data, such as blood pressure and heart rate; subjective data such as previous injury history is also recorded. This is critical for ascertaining the current state of readiness and where the client will start after initial fitness consultations.

Here are six components of a practical movement assessment:
- **Intake of Client**
- **Static Postural Assessment**
- **Assessment of Overhead Squat**
- **Split leg and Single Leg Assessment**
- **Assessment on loaded**
- **Assessment on dynamics**

Before we start, though, let's go over some important aspects of the movement assessment process.

Movement Assessment

In designing an all-encompassing program, knowing how well your client moves is a very crucial piece of information. While conducting my doctoral research, It became evident that many trainers did not use the information gotten from corrective exercise movement assessments.

They often time resulted in using techniques they preferred even after gathering so much information on their clients, not minding if using the information gathered helped their client better. This situation is known as "analysis paralysis," or being unable to make a decision because of information overload. Movement assessments should adhere to a process or flow. This process should prioritize obtaining the most usable amount of information possible, with minimal risk, in the shortest amount of time first. The final part is vital because it shows that not every detail gotten from a single activity can be applied to all clients.

A pro should

be able to conduct a movement assessment flow or process easily. It should be arranged logically, and we should be able to use the information from one test to inform the next test. Further, a client's emotions should be considered as a personal trainer goes through the assessments. The last thing a personal trainer wants his client to feel is that they are not cut out for exercise because they cannot effectively use their motor skills like they used to. Use movement assessments, but make sure to use them intelligently.

They are a starting point for creating a personalized movement assessment flow. The information given here is established on years of experience and logic, but you may vary your test flow based on your environment, client, and training.

INTAKE OF CLIENT

Before we carry out any assessments or movement tests, the personal trainer should interview the client to determine their goals and objectives. This is vital because if a client's main goal is to stand up off the couch and walk a short distance every day, there may be no need to put them through advanced testing. Client intake also counts completing the Physical Activity Readiness Questionnaire (PAR-Q), which will reveal any medical conditions or other reasons why exercise should not be performed. If all is fine, move to step 2.

- **STATIC POSTURAL ASSESSMENT**

The Static Postural Assessment is a picture of a client's posture without movement. Here, the fit pro will pay attention to the five kinetic chain checkpoints (KCC), including the knee, foot and ankle, LPHC, shoulders and thoracic spine, and head and neck. The fit pro should match this to what is considered "ideal" posture (i.e., everything in alignment).

For example, in some cases, severe forward rounding of the shoulders may be the last step before programming begins. By critically monitoring someone's static posture, we can have an accurate idea of which muscles need flexibility and muscles that require strengthening. You can proceed to step three of the Fit pro deems the client fit enough.

2. OVERHEAD SQUAT ASSESSMENT (OHSA)

The OHSA is our first authentic look at movement. It reveals how well the client can control their average range of motion, movement, stability, and coordination. If a client is unable to squat, it may not indicate a musculoskeletal wreck about to happen.

Instead, the lack of ability may be a lack of proper understanding. So, if a client that you presume is somewhat competent performing below expectations, encourage them using tips such as "assume you are sitting in a chair" or "nice job on that first one, let's see if you can keep your feet a little straighter."

You can also give them an actual chair to sit on. Making the assessment, something done every day, will provide a clear view of this movement pattern. Also, just because some people compensate does not mean they are terrible people.

A trainer should take notes and apply them to the program rather than pointing out the failures of the clients.

Next, if the client exhibits signs of compensations of feet turn out, knee valgus, or extreme forward lean, shift to the heels elevated modification – 3 (a). If the client exhibits signs of anterior pelvic tilt (APT) compensation, then use the hands-on-hips modification – 3 (b).

3 (A). HEELS ELEVATED MODIFICATION

This will have the client place their hands on their hips and re-attempt the squat. This modification gets rid of the latissimus dorsi.

If the APT gets better, then the lats are likely the basis causes, and therefore the fit pro could either move forward with shoulder mobility testing or if they feel confident, attempt rolling and stretching the lats. In a case where placing the hands on the hips does not help the APT improve, something particular to the hip complex might be the root cause of the compensation.

A lot of times, the movement assessment process may end here. If the client demonstrated compensations and, therefore, the fit pro has enough information to design a program that will improve the pattern and help the client reach their goals, no additional testing is necessary.

However, if no compensation is present within the OHSA or if the fit pro believes the client can handle more advanced testing and therefore the additional information is warranted, move on to step 4.

- **SINGLE-LEG SQUAT ASSESSMENT (SLSA) OR SPLIT SQUAT ASSESSMENT (SSA)**

Present the client with two options based on ability. If competent (i.e., the fit pro has cause to assume that the client can safely perform the single-leg squat), then have the client do the SLSA. However, if not competent (i.e., the fit pro has reason to assume that the client will not be entirely safe in a single-leg attempt), then have the client do the SSA.

The SSA is seen just like the SLSA, from the front and primarily exploring knee and pelvic stability. During the SSA, direct the client to keep a toe on the ground for additional support. The trainer needs to keep in mind which toe the client uses so the reassessment will be valid.

A personal trainer may bring an end to the assessments at this point and move to training sessions depending on the client and their goals. Sufficient information on overall movement ability can be provided by these 4–6 (including modifications) assessments and point out which muscles may be a little weak and which may be a little short.

However, if after the four previous assessments, fit pro thinks more advanced movement assessments will produce additional usable information, then they should proceed to the "optional" Loaded Assessment (step 5) and/or the Dynamic Assessments (step 6).

2. LOADED ASSESSMENTS

Loaded assessments are simply what the name indicates: a loaded movement that the fit pro adds as part of the assessment. However, the client should not be allowed to know that this is a continuous assessment and should treat this assessment as part of the actual workout.

For Loaded Assessments, the fit pro should create a program that monitors the primary movement patterns, such as squats, lunges, hinges, pushes, and pulls. The personal trainer should not use too much weight on each. Select a reasonable weight and monitor how the client handles it.

Watch for any breaks in form, inability to have controlled breath during the movements, or inconsistency in form. One thing to consider is that a client might break down while loaded and do well while not loaded. This may be due to a strength or stability issue versus short and overactive muscles.

3. DYNAMIC ASSESSMENTS

Dynamic Assessments should be used for clients with higher levels of coordination, control, and stability and those with performance-specific goals. While there is a range of dynamic assessments to choose from, NASM recommends at least one for lower- and one for the upper-extremities.

For the upper extremity, we propose the Davies Test as it is easy to perform and gives excellent insight into the clients' ability to stabilize and control the upper body. For lower extremities, the Depth Jump Assessment is easy to execute and produces sufficient data for programming.

Movement assessments give a wide range of data that is required to create an individualized program. Notwithstanding, given the range of available movement assessments, it may be difficult to know when and why to carry out a test.

As earlier stated, all fit pros need to find what techniques work best for them, taking into account their environment and specific clientele. However, make sure all tests have their purpose and do not just "go through the motions." If the information obtained is not going to aid the programming, then do not waste the client's time.

Here's a quick recap for you.

- **Start by interviewing your clients** and doing the basic physical activity readiness questionnaire to appraise overall movements from a purely preliminary standpoint.

- **Proceed to a Static Postural Assessment** by observing the five kinetic checkpoints (KCC), including the LPHC, foot and ankle, knee, shoulders and thoracic spine, and head and neck.
- **The Overhead Squat Assessment** is the primary overall look at any client movement. With heels elevated and hands-on-hip modifications, this assessment can serve as useful windows into the client's overall movement health.
- **Single-Leg and Split-Squat assessments come next.** Depending on the client's ability, you can bring the assessment to an end here, and your client movement knowledge would still be sufficient.
- **Loaded Assessments** are more advanced and need assessing movements when the client has weights. Lack of strength and coordination might result in a breakdown in form and the introduction of movement compensations instead of underactive or overactive muscles.
- **Dynamic Assessments** are also for more advanced movement analysis and are geared towards performance-related fitness metrics.

Practice Questions

- **Of all the following muscles, only one is not overactive in upper crossed syndrome. Which?**

A. levator scapulae
B. upper trapezius
C. deep cervical flexors
D. sternocleidomastoid

Answer:

The Correct Answer to the question is 'C'. deep cervical flexors

This is due to the fact that the deep cervical flexors belong to the lower body region, also known as the pelvic girdle. Hence, it can be subject to the lower crossed syndrome. Also, all other options are subject to the shoulder girdle upper crossed syndrome.

2. When wearing shoes with high heels, what position is the ankle put in?

A. dorsi flexed position
B. a pronated position
C. a supinated position
D. a plantar flexed position

Answer:

The Correct Answer to the question is 'D'. a plantar flexed position

In a position like this, the heel is raised and as a result, sufficient force is fed through the forefoot. This is always due to the shortening of the calf muscles. The main muscles are called the soleus and gastrocnemius. And since the Dorsi means upwards flex, the heeled shoes would therefore force a downward flex. The other options with bothers on pronation and supination simply talks about the way up the body or the way the body part is oriented.

3. In the upper crossed syndrome, which joint mechanic is present?
A. Increased scapular protraction
B. Increased shoulder extension
C. Increased shoulder rotation
D. Decreased cervical extension

Answer:

The Correct Answer to the question is 'A'. Increased scapular protraction

Upper crossed syndrome deals with the shoulder girdle. That rules out B, cervical extension, which would apply to the pelvic girdle. Cross syndrome refers to imbalances occurring across the midline which means C and D, extension, and rotation do not apply, leaving only A.

4. The Durnin formula includes all of the following skinfold sites except:
A. Triceps
B. Subscapular.
C. Midaxillary
D. Biceps

Answer:

The Correct Answer is C. Midaxillary

Midaxillary is an anatomical line and not a site on the body which one can take skinfold measurements from.

5. What assessment is good for the single leg squat assessment?
A. Overhead squat assessment
B. Inline lunge assessment
C. Single-leg balance assessment
D. Stork balance test

Answer:

The Correct Answer to the question is 'C'. Single-leg balance assessment

Since the single leg squat assessment is engaged on just one unsupported leg, the single-leg balance assessment is the closest approximation to it. While the stork balance test is also conducted on a single leg, it is however conducted by supporting the standing leg with the raised leg.

6. For what reason is the L.E.F.T. test conducted?
A. L.E.F.T. assesses dexterity, acceleration, and deceleration
B. L.E.F.T. assesses speed, explosive power, and neuromuscular regulation
C. L.E.F.T. assesses dynamic posture, lower extremity power, and speed
D. L.E.F.T. assesses gait, body control, speed, and balance

Answer:

The Correct Answer is A. L.E.F.T. assesses dexterity, acceleration, and deceleration

L.E.F.T. is an agility assessment. Agility consists of dexterity, acceleration, and deceleration. While D might seem like a sensible choice, speed, explosive power, and neuromuscular regulation are not exclusive to agility.

7. If you have a 45-year-old client who is healthy but sedentary, and such client has been instructed by the doctor to increase flexibility and build

some muscle via exercise, what are the best collective of assessment objectives you would prescribe as a personal trainer?

A. Circumference measurements, Step Test, Overhead squat assessment, Push-Up Test, Shark Skill Test, Upper extremity strength assessment
B. Body fat measurement, Step Test, Davies Test, Shark Skill Test, Lower extremity strength assessment
C. Medical release from the client's physician, Resting heart rate, Blood pressure, Step Test, Overhead squat assessment, Assisted single-leg squat assessment
D. Body fat measurement, Circumference measurements, Resting heart rate, Blood pressure, Step Test, Overhead squat assessment, Single-leg balance/squat

Answer:

The Correct Answer is D. Body fat measurement, Circumference measurements, Resting heart rate, Blood pressure, Step Test, Overhead squat assessment, Single-leg balance/squat

Body fat measurements and circumference measurements will allow the trainer to determine the client's recommended weight loss strategy. Resting heart rate, blood pressure, and step test will assess for potential exercise readiness risk factors with regards to cardiac health. Lastly, the squat assessments will determine how capable she will be regarding her previous knee injury.

8. Which of these are cardiorespiratory assessments?
A. Rockport Walk Test and Davies Test
B. YMCA 3-Minute Step Test and Rockport Walk Test
C. Davies Test and Shark Skill Test
D. YMCA 3-Minute Step Test and Davies Test

Answer:

The Correct Answer is B. YMCA 3-Minute Step Test and Rockport Walk Test

Both these drills are designed to assess cardiorespiratory readiness. The Davies Test and Shark Test are used to assess strength performance, this rules out all options that include the Davies test.

9. What signifies a lower resting heart rate?
A. A less efficient and fit cardiorespiratory system
B. Overtraining or increased life stress
C. Poor sleeping patterns
D. A more efficient and fit cardiorespiratory system

Answer:

The Correct Answer is D. A more efficient and fit cardiorespiratory system

A lower resting heart rate is significant for improved health and quality of life which includes having an optimized cardiorespiratory system.

10. Of all the options, which muscle becomes overactive when a person is demonstrating an excessive forward lean?
A. Gastrocnemius
B. Anterior tibialis
C. Gluteus maximus
D. Erector spinae

Answer:

The Correct Answer is A. Gastrocnemius

An overactive gastrocnemius can lead to forwarding lean, noticeable during a squat assessment. This could also be due to tight soleus and hip flexors, but based on available options, the Correct Answer to the question is A.

Chapter 4

Program Design

The Program Design domain is meant to evaluate a candidate's ability to use assessment results to create appropriate exercise programs for individual clients, including flexibility training, core training, resistance training, balance training, cardiorespiratory training, and plyometric and speed coordination speed training.

The program design is the meal of being a successful fitness trainer. In lieu of this, NASM has made program drawing the second most focused domain of the lot. It does not fall behind the number one spot.

The largest part of the NASM Program Design is the **OPT model or optimal performance training**. A strong understanding of periodization will also count in your favor.

Other areas of focus consist

- **Operation systems (GAS, SAID, Overload, Variation)**
- **Periodization methodologies (linear, undulating)**
- **latest trends**

The Optimum Performance Training Model

Exercise programs need individuality, based on the client's assessment results, to make them impactful for clients, which likely increases adherence to the program. Exercise programs must consider many variables, such as teaching proper movement patterns, improving mobility and stability, enhancing endurance, and reducing the likelihood of injury. A training plan determines the forms of training to be used, how long it will take, how often it will change, and what will perform specifically. A periodization is a systematic approach to program design that varies the amount and type of stress placed on the body to produce a physical adaptation and reduce the likelihood of overtraining and injury.

An annual training plan, or macrocycle, demonstrates the long-term training program. A weekly schedule, or microcycle, describes the distinct workouts. Linear periodization gradually increases the training program's intensity while simultaneously decreasing volume over a particular period. Undulating periodization uses changes in volume, power, and exercise selection to provide loading differences daily or weekly.

The OPT model consists of three levels: stabilization, strength, and power.

The OPT model includes five distinctive phases of training:
- **Phase 1 Stabilization Endurance Training**
- **Phase 2 Strength Endurance Training**
- **Phase 3 Muscular Development Training**
- **Phase 4 Maximal Strength Training**
- **Phase 5 Power Training**

The OPT workout template is divided into six parts: Warm-up, Activation, Skill Development, Resistance Training, Client Choice, and Cool-down. Can integrate Cardiorespiratory training into any section of the OPT template.

Phase 1: Stabilization Endurance Training teaches clients how to perform proper
movement patterns, including pushing, pulling, pressing, squatting, hip hinging, trunk
rotation, and overall movement competency. Once clients display good movement patterns, Phase 1 programs are progressed by emphasizing enhancing proprioception, balance, and postural control.

Phase 2: Strength Endurance Training is a hybrid form of training that involves superset training. A stabilization-focused practice immediately follows a strength-focused exercise with similar biomechanical motions.

Phase 3: Muscular Development Training is designed to enhance muscle hypertrophy using a high volume of strength-focused exercises.

Phase 4: Maximal Strength Training requires the inclusion of heavy resistance training exercises to increase muscular strength.

Phase 5: Power Training uses superset techniques to increase the rate of force production. These superset techniques include performing a heavy resistance training exercise followed by an explosive power-based exercise with similar biomechanical motions.

The OPT model is an exercise program model that uses both linear and undulating periodization to help clients of all levels and abilities achieve a variety of different goals, including but not limited to reduced body fat, increased muscle mass, and improved athletic performance.

NASM Endorsement For Program Design

To increase the work process, NASM suggests that fitness coaches should create a coordinated method to it. coordinated training includes multiple forms of exercise such as flexibility, cardiorespiratory; core; balance; plyometrics, speed, agility, and quickness (SAQ); and resistance training.

Using a coordinated approach to program design can increase consistency and progression and minimize injury risk. upholding these, the most important factor when creating a program is to make sure it is adopted and strictly carried out by the trainee.

These attributes increase commitment and help sustain a client's success towards achieving their fitness desires. These are the initial stages of NASM's Optimum Performance Training (OPT) model, its recent updates, and refurbished procedures.

Why did NASM Design OPT?

The OPT model is a organized training program with precise planning, system, and periodic assessment. It is designed to improve the physical abilities and mental coordination simultaneously. Undergoing the OPT model can boost your balance, core stability, aerobic endurance, flexibility, and muscular build-up. Over the years, the system has proven to be highly successful in helping clients and athletes from diverse populations reduce their body fat, increase lean muscle mass, and improve athletic performance and overall health.

The OPT program is majorly divided into three levels, stabilization, strength, and power, and is further subdivided into five phases. Each phase has specific protocols, exercise guidelines, and acute variables (i.e., sets, repetitions, rest periods, etc.).

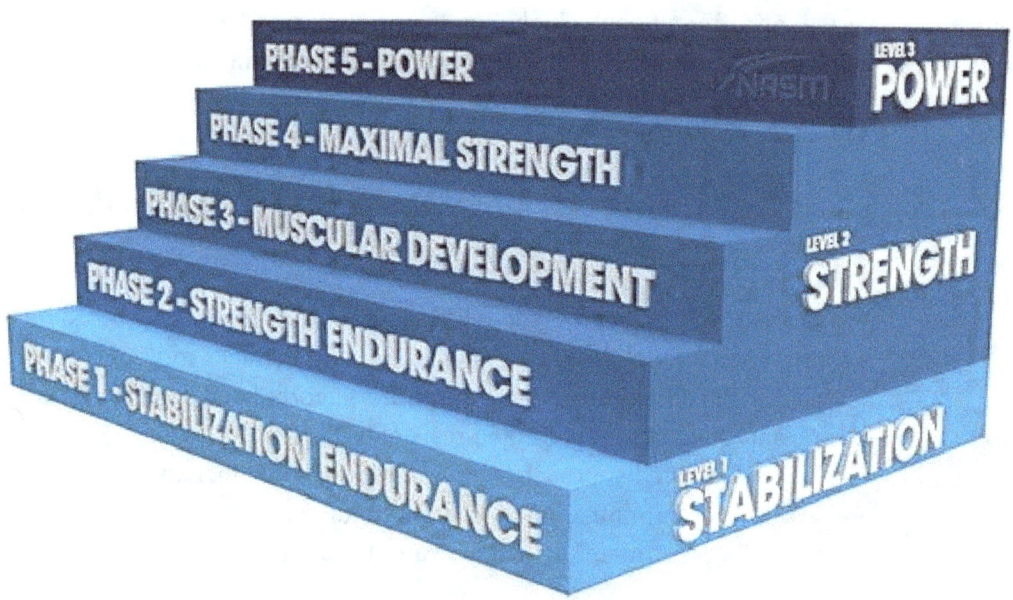

The OPT model should be considered a staircase, guiding clients through different physical adaptation levels as shown in the above table. This will involve going up and down the stairs, stopping at other steps, and moving to various heights; it depends on what the client wants to achieve.

Table 1 Summary Chart of the OPT Model

Level	Phase	Primary Adaptations	Primary Methods of Progression
Stabilization	1. Stabilization Endurance Training	· Movement and flexibility · Major and joint stabilization · Postural alignment and control · Muscular and aerobic endurance	· Progress exercises proprioceptively (controlled, yet unstable) · Increase the complexity of exercises once basic movement patterns have been established.

Strength	2. Strength Endurance Training	· Core strength and joint stabilization · Muscular endurance and prime mover strength	· Decrease rest periods. · Increase the volume of exercises (reps + sets). · Increase the load (weight) of resistance training exercises. · Increase the complexity of resistance training exercises.
	3. Hypertrophy Training (Muscular Growth Training)	· macular strength · Muscular energy and hypertrophy	· Improve the volume of exercises. · Improve the load of resistance training exercises. · Improve the complexity of resistance training exercises.

	3. Hypertrophy Training (Muscular Growth Training)	· macular strength · Muscular energy and hypertrophy	· Improve the volume of exercises. · Improve the load of resistance training exercises. · Improve the complexity of resistance training exercises.
	4. Highest Strength training	· major strength · Highest muscular strength	· Improve the load of resistance training exercises. · Improve the sets of resistance training exercises.
	3. Hypertrophy Training (Muscular Growth Training)	· macular strength · Muscular energy and hypertrophy	· Improve the volume of exercises. · Improve the load of resistance training exercises. · Improve the complexity of resistance training exercises.

	4. Highest Strength training	· major strength · Highest muscular strength	· Improve the load of resistance training exercises. · Improve the sets of resistance training exercises.
	P5. Power activity	· Major strength · highest muscular energy · value of energy production	· Improve the load of resistance training exercises. · Improve the speed (repetition tempo) of exercises. · Improve the sets of exercises.

The NASM 2020 Optima Conference revealed new guidelines and protocols for the OPT model. These guidelines reflect the recent scientific discovery and feedback from many people, such as; academicians, researchers, and practitioners, to increase client outcomes and adherence to exercise programs. New OPT guidelines reflect five primary outcomes:

1. Emphasis on training fundamental movement patterns.
2. New warm-up protocols.
3. Integrate corrective exercise.
4. Less rigidity and more creative choice.
5. Inclusion of behavior change techniques.

Fundamental Patterns for Movement Training

Fundamental movement patterns are essential for all fitness coaches so as to show and train their clients. Fitness coaches must see to it that their trainees master these movement patterns to reduce injury risk and maximize training strength.

However, multiple movement patterns can be combined into a single exercise, such as squatting, hip hinge, pulling motions, pushing motions, pressing, and multiplanar and rotational movement.

As a result, attention to training fundamental movement patterns has been added to Phase 1 of the OPT Model.

A popular example is a client moving utilizing selected equipment to barbells, dumbbells, and other forms of free-weights.

New Warm-Up Protocols

New research has come forth as touching warm-up and stretching protocols. Normally, stage 1 includes self-myofascial techniques and static stretching, whereas stage 2-4 opted for self-myofascial techniques and active stretching, and stage 5 used self-myofascial techniques and dynamic stretching (no static or active stretching. Despite this, based on the new guidelines, fitness professionals can now include dynamic stretching in all OPT model phases.

The addition of dynamic stretches may further add joint range of motion in the process, also adding to the potential expression of strength and energy output. If choosing to include dynamic stretching, choose one set of 3-10 flexible stretches using a repetition range of 10 to 15.

Table 2 Warm-up Protocols			
Level	**Phase**	**Original Warm-up Protocol**	**Revised Warm-up Protocol**

Stabilization	Phase 1.	· Self-myofascial Techniques · Static Stretching · Cardio (optional)	· Self-myofascial Techniques · Static Stretching · Dynamic Stretching (optional) · Cardio (optional)
Strength	Phases 2-4	· Self-myofascial Techniques · Static Stretching · Cardio (optional)	· Self-myofascial methods · Static Stretching · Dynamic Stretching (optional) · Cardio (optional)
Power	Phase 5	· Self-myofascial me · Dynamic Stretching	· Self-myofascial Techniques · Dynamic Stretching

Integrate Corrective Exercise Protocols

Every phase of training, OPT model recommends the use of major and balanced training due to the warm-ups. This section of the training is a continuation of the client's overall introduction. The client addressed overactive muscles in the warm-up area by performing various flexibility to improve range movement and tissue capability.

The next reasonable step is to strengthen the underactive muscles identified during the assessment process, helping reestablish ideal joint alignment, stability, and control. Can accomplish this by completing a short series of core and balance activities. Core training is critical for improving posture, enhancing performance, increasing resistance to injury, and accelerating injury rehabilitation. Balance training is an important part of injury preventive measures of the training and has been certified to help reduce the incidence of lower extremity injuries, such as ankle sprains and anterior cruciate ligament tears. As such, major and balance training, when paired, can be a useful warm-up strategy that follows flexible methods.

In addition, fitness coaches are people with knowledge and skills in workouts that may replace other methods. In this section, such isolated strengthening methods taught in NASM's Corrective fitness Specialist. Endorsing isolated strengthening techniques into an OPT Model exercise program effectively combines corrective exercise and OPT.

The coach typically assigns plyometric and speed, agility, and quickness (SAQ) exercises within this section. This type of exercise further enhances energy expenditure and creates personal skill, reaction time, and overall athleticism. Also, plyometric and SAQ training are important ways of training to increase aerobic strength and can also be used as a substitute for traditional steady-state cardiorespiratory exercise if they think it is necessary.

Besides, fitness coaches also can forego plyometric and SAQ exercises, choosing to substitute specialized instruction for skill acquisition. For example, can include education for specialized exercise equipment (i.e., kettlebells, battle ropes) in this part of the workout te
technique.

For very advanced trainees, the fitness coach can teach new skills which include; practicing MMA-inspired exercises (e.g., kicking and punching a bag), acquiring knowledge on the intricacies of Olympic weightlifting, or integrating mind-body movements (e.g., Pilates, yoga, tai chi). It is important to identify that any exercises chosen in this section by the fitness professional should be based on the trainee's visible strength, goals, and exercise preferences.

Optimum Performance Training® — NASM

CLIENT'S NAME:					
GOAL:					
PHASE:					
DATE:					
EXERCISE	SETS	REPS	TEMPO	REST	NOTES
WARM-UP					
ACTIVATION (core & balance)					
SKILL DEVELOPMENT (plyometric & SAQ)					
RESISTANCE TRAINING					
CLIENT'S CHOICE					
COOL-DOWN					

Coaching Tips:

Introduction of Techniques For Behavior Change

The most vital thing to consider when making exercise outlines is to make sure that clients adhere to it. A fitness coach can influence clients' health, body composition, and athletic performance. In lieu of this, the fitness professional has a responsibility to make an area that h the client adheres to a fitness routine. They should motivate clients while preserving their independence to do the exercises they prefer. Self-efficacy is a well-established determinant.

In this section, the trainee chooses a few of their favorite exercises to include in the program.

Introduction to Exercise Modalities

Exercise modalities are tools that are designed to enhance an exercise or movement to create a desired outcome. There are many types of exercise modalities, including resistance training equipment, balance tools, and fitness trackers.

It is important to keep safety and effectiveness in mind when deciding which training modalities may be the best to use and when to integrate them into a program. Because most novice exercisers lack resistance training experience, strength-training machines may offer a safer and effective option to free weights. Strength-training machines, however, are regarded as inferior to free weights for improving core stability and muscular coordination, as they offer artificial support instead of using one's core
musculature. A large population can use free weights, in a variety of fashions, for many goals and in all phases of the OPT model. Although extremely versatile, free weights can be intimidating.
Cable machines can provide greater ROM when compared to selectorized strength equipment. When using cable machines, it is important to match the cable's resistance to the muscle's natural line of pull.
 Elastic bands and tubing also allow clients to perform resisted exercises that mimic sport-specific movements, such as a golf swing or tennis forehand. Elastic resistance is portable and inexpensive but may not be ideal when trying to develop high levels of strength and muscular hypertrophy.

Medicine balls can be used like other resistance implements to add load or instability to an exercise. Medicine balls can be used with a variety of populations as part of a program to increase muscular strength, endurance, and power, or in some cases, to help rehabilitate from injury. A kettlebell is not the same with a dumbbell, barbell, or medicine ball because the center of mass is far away from the handle, which may demand more energy and focus, as well as increased recruitment from stabilizers and young movers simultaneously during specific movements. Many kettlebell exercises involve multiple joint motions and muscle groups.

Suspended bodyweight training is an innovative approach to bodyweight fitness training in that it uses a system called a system of ropes and webbing that allows the user to work against their own body weight while performing various exercises. Sandbags are designed to be carried, lifted, thrown, and pulled, and most come with several handles to easily change grips. Unlike barbells, dumbbells, and selectorized machines, the sand within the bag is constantly shifting, providing continuous instability. ViPR is an acronym for vitality, performance, and reconditioning. It is designed to be dragged, tossed, lifted, pulled, pressed, and carried. This design allows the fitness professional to perform multidirectional, full-body exercises with external load resistance, known as loaded movement training.

Battle ropes are typically made of heavy-duty nylon and come in a variety of lengths and thicknesses. Battle ropes are low-impact activities, which provide less impact on the joints. Balance modalities improve balance, ankle stability, and coordination but should not perform maximal or near-maximal lifts for safety reasons. Stability balls, also known as Swiss balls, are popularly used in various training facilities with a wide range of populations. They are basically used to increase the demand for stability in an exercise and use them to reinforce proper posture during squatting movements.

The BOSU ball is an inflated rubber area tied to a solid plastic surface; it looks like a stability ball cut in half. Training with the BOSU ball offers the opportunity to increase the intensity of an exercise by decreasing the stability. The Terra-Core consists of an inflatable rubber bladder and hard-surfaced backing. Unlike stability balls, it is safe to perform several resistance training exercises, such as a dumbbell chest press, while lying supine on the Terra-Core.

Fitness trackers are electronic wearable devices that enable a user to track their activity levels. They come in many forms, such as watches, bands, rings, heart rate monitors, and pedometers. Ease of use and intrinsic motivation are key factors for continued fitness trackers among those who purchase trackers.

Chronic Health Conditions and Special Populations

There is a significant need for increased awareness and access to general fitness training for youths year-round, not just during one or more sports seasons. Due to the overwhelming increase in childhood obesity and diabetes, current youth fitness guidelines focus on promoting healthy lifestyles and health-related physical fitness.

The latest recommendations state that children and adolescents should get 60 minutes (1 hour) or more of moderate to vigorous bodily activity daily. It is, therefore, crucial to understand that there are fundamental physiologic differences between children and adults. Research has demonstrated that resistance training is both safe and effective in children and adolescents.

Despite the normal decline in physiologic functioning associated with aging, older adults—with and without other chronic health conditions—can respond to exercise much in the same manner as apparently healthy younger adults. By adhering to a systematic process, fitness professionals can dramatically impact the overall health and well-being of older adults. Regular physical activity and exercise are some of the most important factors related to long-term successful weight loss.

Exercise has been shown to have a substantial positive effect on the treatment and prevention of type 2 diabetes. Clients with stable coronary artery disease—especially those who have participated in a cardiac rehabilitation programs—should know or be taught information on the importance and benefits of exercise, which includes a lower risk of mortality, increased exercise tolerance, muscle strength, reduction in angina and heart failure symptoms, and improved psychological status and social adjustment.

Exercise regimens that combine resistance training to increase BMD with flexibility, core, and balance training to enhance proprioception are important for clients with osteoporosis and osteopenia. Fitness professionals need to understand the difference between rheumatoid arthritis and osteoarthritis and be aware of the signs and symptoms of an acute rheumatoid arthritis exacerbation. Fitness professionals should also monitor clients' progress with arthritis to assess the effects of the exercise program on joint pain. Exercise is an important intervention for clients recovering from cancer. It can improve exercise tolerance, reduce the cellular risks associated with cancer, and improve quality of life.

There has been tangible research documenting the beneficial effects of exercise during pregnancy on the physiology and health of both the mother and developing fetus. Clients with lung disease experience fatigue at low levels of activity and often experience dyspnea. The primary limiting factor for training in the client with PAD is leg pain. making and modifying exercise programs for clients can be complicated because many variables are considered, including the client's goals, exercise tolerance, and unique physical abilities, and medical history

Practice Questions

- **Why do we consider slower tempos for stabilization and patience?**

A. The tempo activates less weakness and longer energy
B. The rate is inversely related to training strength
C. The velocity is inhibited by the strength of the trainee
D. The slow movement improves nervous system preparation time

Answer:

The Correct Answer to the question is 'D'. The slow movement improves nervous system preparation time.

To achieve a good level of endurance and stability gains, the time under tension is required in order to properly stimulate optimization. This would be done via improved nervous system adaptation.

2. What makes performance improve when they are within sets?
A. Adenine and cytosine are minimized during training, and rest allows replenishment
B. Glutamine and tyrosine are minimized during training, and rest allows replenishment
C. Methionine and adenosine triphosphate are minimized during training, and rest allows replenishment
D. Adenosine triphosphate and phosphocreatine are minimized during exercise, and rest allows replenishment

Answer:

The Correct Answer to the question is 'D'. Adenosine triphosphate and phosphocreatine are minimized during exercise, and rest allows replenishment.

The cycling between ATP and ADP is very effective over a limited time span. After this, a brief cooldown is required for ADP and creative levels to re-calibrate so as to produce an optimal amount of energy.

3. Which rep range is best for maximal force modification?
A. 1 to 10 reps at 30 to 45% 1RM
B. 1 to 5 reps at 85 to 100% 1RM
C. 12 to 20 reps at 50 to 70% 1RM
D. 6 to 12 reps at 75 to 85% 1RM

Answer:

The Correct Answer to the question is 'B'. 1 to 5 reps at 85-100% 1RM

Maximal strength is produced at the highest intensity and lowest volume possible. 'B' is ideal for hypertrophy with limited strength adaptations, while A and Clean more towards the endurance-based adaptations.

4. Which of these produces hypertrophy and fat loss?
A. High volume, low/moderate-intensity training
B. Low volume, maximal strength training
C. Low volume, high-intensity training
D. High volume, high-intensity training

Answer:

The Correct Answer is A. High volume, low/moderate-intensity training

For fat loss to occur, metabolic stress needs to be achieved during training. For hypertrophy to occur, mechanical stress needs to be achieved during training. For the two to occur simultaneously, the best option is A, which is a compromise of the high volume for optimal fat loss and high intensity for optimal hypertrophy.

5. Why should we not discontinue stabilization training both during and after energy and power workout?
A. Stabilization training is the most thorough cardiorespiratory exercise
B. Stabilization training will consume more calories
C. Stabilization training will increase the rate of force production
D. Stabilisation exercise will keep major and joint stability

Answer:

The Correct Answer to the question is 'D'. Stabilization training will keep major and joint stability.

Having well-conditioned stability of the core and joints is necessary for sustained and progressive training over the long and short term. A and B are not directly influenced by stabilization training, and C is a byproduct of good adaptation, helped in part, but not directly by stabilization.

6. Which of these is not a low-volume training adaptation?
A. Increased rate of force production
B. Increased cross-sectional muscle area
C. Increased motor unit recruitment
D. Increased motor unit synchronization

Answer:

The Correct Answer is B. Increased cross-sectional muscle area.

A high volume, low to moderate intensity protocol is required for an increase in muscle cross-sectional area. A, C, and D are all adaptations of low-volume training.

7. How much of our ATP and phosphocreatine is it possible to gain in 20-30 seconds?
A. 100%
B. 50%

C. 75%
D. 85%

Answer:
The Correct Answer is B. 50%

In order to replenish ATP and creatine stores to full capacity, a required restoration period of between 7 to 10 mins is necessary. Because the rate of replenishment diminishes over time, the ATP-PC stocks will bounce back to 50% in relatively little time but will take increasingly longer to fill up more.

8. Which of these sets, reps, intensity, tempo, and rest do you think support power exercise?
A. 1-5, 3-6, 30-45% 1RM, fast/explosive, 0 to 60 sec
B. 1-10, 3-6, 85-100% 1RM, fast/explosive, 3 to 5 min
C. 1-5, 4-6, 85-100% 1RM, fast/explosive, 3 to 5 min
D. 1-10, 3-6, 30-45% 1RM, fast/explosive, 3 to 5 min

Answer:

The Correct Answer to the question is D'. 1-10, 3-6, 30-45% 1RM, fast/explosive, 3-5 minutes

All options check out when it comes to tempo. That's because power training or plyometric training is an attempt to engage maximal force production over as short a period of time as possible by decreasing the amortization phase. All options also check our regarding rest interval except for A.

Adequate rest is required in order to replenish ATP phosphocreatine levels to a point where they can supply enough energy for maximum output in each set. The intensity required for power training is much lower than for strength and even hypertrophy. Since A is not an option based on rest, and B and C are not eligible due to intensity, it leaves D as the correct choice.

9. Which is not a multi-joint exercise?
A. Calf raises
B. Squats

C. Step-ups
D. Chest presses

Answer:

The Correct Answer is A. Calf raises

This question is confusing because most people assume the practitioner to be using multiple joints in all exercises. A calf raise in this case would be said to be multi-joint due to the engagement of both calves. The question refers to a variety of joints used as opposed to an upfront number, of which the only calf raises uses one variety, the ankle.

10. Which rep tempo is perfect for increasing muscular endurance and stabilization?
A. 4/2/1
B. 1/4/1
C. 1/0/1
D. 2/0/2

Answer:

The Correct Answer to the question is 'A'. 4/2/1

To provide the required time under tension, a longer tempo is ideal. This will help stimulate endurance adaptations. Also, a longer tempo can provide the nervous system with the opportunity to prepare.

Chapter 5

Exercise Techniques and Training Instruction

The Exercise Technique and Training Instruction is designed to measure the candidate's ability and knowledge of effective and safe exercise techniques, correct set-up and technique of various exercises and training methods, proper spotting techniques, warm-up and cool-down protocols, safe training practices, cueing techniques, kinetic chain checkpoints, and signs indicating that training modifications are needed.

This is the most eminent domain in the exam, but only by a single percentage. Here you will get the chance to be tested on your ability as a coach in real-time, facing real-world scenarios. Your knowledge and capacity to identify and execute proper exercise protocols and forms of techniques will also be assessed. The goal is to optimize your capability to produce results and accomplish them safely.

Concentrate on all the major training methodologies such as SAQ, flexibility, resistance, core training, and balance. You will also need an understanding of different types of equipment and apparatus you can employ for exercise instruction, and successfully group different exercises based on which training methodology they fall under.

Focus on the various training methodology charts, understand the modalities, and know by heart a few exercises in each category.

Other points of focus include:
- **Cueing techniques (kinesthetic, visual, and auditory)**
- **Exercise regression and progression**
- **Spotting techniques**

Integrated Training and the OPT Model

Integrated training combines flexibility, cardiorespiratory, core, balance, plyometrics, SAQ, and resistance training into one system. When an exercise program is progressive and systematic, using a progressive overload approach, the body becomes stronger by adapting to the new demands placed on it. Fundamental movement patterns include squatting, hip hinge, pulling, pushing, and pressing.

Maintaining ideal posture places the client's body in the most optimal state to perform movement patterns safely and effectively. Optimal ROM allows joints to move freely. Fitness professionals should provide programming that requires movement in all three planes of motion: sagittal, frontal, and transverse. The acute variables for training include repetitions, sets, training intensity, repetition tempo, rest interval, training volume, training frequency, training duration, exercise selection, and exercise order.

An ever-changing integrated training approach provides a systematic and progressive approach to fitness training; its components include flexibility, cardiorespiratory, core, balance, plyometric (reactive), SAQ, and resistance training. Benefits of flexibility training include increased joint ROM, a possible decrease in muscle soreness, and a potential reduction in injury risk. Benefits of cardiorespiratory training include decreased heart rate and blood pressure while increasing stroke volume and cardiac output.

Benefits of core training include enhanced posture; better bodily function for daily living; increased balance, stabilization, and coordination of the kinetic chain; minimized low-back pain, and improved skill-related movements. Benefits of balance training include reducing the risk of falls and ankle sprains while improving proprioception and agility-based activities.

Plyometric (reactive) training benefits include improved bone mineral density and soft tissue strength, expression of power, and explosiveness while also increasing metabolic expenditures required for weight management.

Benefits of SAQ training include improved top speed, change in direction, and rate of acceleration and deceleration. Benefits of resistance training include increased endurance, strength, and power; muscular hypertrophy; and weight management. The OPT model phases have been properly discussed in the previous chapter. If you missed it, you should go back to check it out.

Flexibility Training Concepts

Flexibility is explained as the normal extensibility of all soft tissues that allow the complete ROM of a joint. Flexibility has a significant influence on mobility during dynamic motion. Relative flexibility can be developed by poor flexibility, which is how the HMS seeks the path of least resistance amidst functional movements.

The HMS, also known as the kinetic chain, comprises the muscular, skeletal, and nervous systems. The body's kinetic chain can be further classified into two regional chains: upper kinetic chain and lower kinetic chain.

Muscle imbalance can be caused by postural distortions, repetitive movement, cumulative trauma, emotional duress, poor training technique, poor bodily control, and biased training patterns. Muscle imbalance may result in altered reciprocal inhibition, synergistic dominance, osteo- and arthrokinematics dysfunction. Synergistic dominance is a neuromuscular phenomenon that occurs when synergists take over function for a weak or inhibited prime mover (agonist). This leads to altered
reciprocal inhibition of the antagonist's muscle. Osteokinematics describes how the bones and joints are moving through a ROM, and arthrokinematics describes the motion at the joint surfaces. Altered muscle length-tension relationships, force-couple relationships, and poor joint surface motion can cause altered joint motion, which results in poor movement efficiency.

Neuromuscular efficiency is the ability of the nervous system to recruit the correct muscles, produce force, reduce force, and dynamically stabilize the body's structure in all three planes of motion. To allow for optimal neuromuscular efficiency, individuals must have good flexibility in all three planes of motion.

The scientific rationale for flexibility training is illustrated through the concept of pattern overload and the cumulative injury cycle. Common types of flexibility exercise include self-myofascial techniques and static, active, and dynamic stretching. Self-myofascial rolling is thought to produce both local mechanical and neurophysiological effects on the myofascial tissues. A process where you passively take a muscle to the point of tension and stay in that form for a minimum of 30 seconds is known as Static stretching.

Active stretching is the process of using agonists and synergists to dynamically move the joint into a ROM, holding for 1 to 2 seconds and repeating for 5 to 10 repetitions. Dynamic stretching uses the force production of a muscle and the body's momentum to take a joint through the full available ROM. Fitness professionals should have a comprehensive understanding of controversial stretches, medical precautions, and contraindications to program a safe flexibility program for clients of all fitness levels.

Cardiorespiratory Fitness Training

Cardiorespiratory fitness shows the ability of the cardiovascular and respiratory systems to supply oxygen-rich blood to skeletal muscles during sustained physical activity. Cardiorespiratory fitness is one of five components of health-related physical fitness; the others include muscular strength, muscular endurance, flexibility, and body composition.

Research has proved that an individual's cardiorespiratory fitness level is a strong predictor of morbidity and mortality. Research demonstrates that cardiorespiratory exercise and physical activity provide many benefits that enhance health, longevity, and weight loss. Cardiorespiratory exercise must be individually determined and should use the FITTE-VP principle. FITTE-VP stands for frequency, intensity, type, time, enjoyment, volume, and progression.

Frequency indicates the number of training sessions in a given period, usually expressed as per week. Moderate-intensity exercise (e.g., brisk walking) should be performed at least five times per week, whereas vigorous-intensity exercise (e.g., jogging or running) should be performed at least three times per week, or a combination of moderate-intensity and vigorous-intensity is also acceptable.

The level of demand that an activity places on the body is called Intensity. Some methods for monitoring cardiorespiratory exercise intensity include calculating O2 max, using percentages of maximal heart rate (HRmax), heart rate reserve (HRR), metabolic equivalents (METs), ratings of perceived exertion (RPE), and the talk test. Time refers to the space of time engaged in an activity or exercise training session and is typically expressed in minutes.

Adults should have a total of 2 hours and 30 minutes (150 minutes) of moderate-intensity aerobic activity this could include brisk walking, every week or an hour and 15 minutes (75 minutes) of vigorous-intensity aerobic activity including jogging or running every week, or a comparable mix of moderate- and vigorous-intensity aerobic activity. Type refers to the mode of activity selected, such as cycling, running, or swimming. Enjoyment indicates the amount of pleasure derived from engaging in a specific exercise or activity.

The volumeThe volume of exercise represents the total amount of work performed in each timeframe, typically one week.
Progression refers to how an exercise program advances. Each exercise training session should also include a warm-up phase, conditioning phase, and cool-down phase.

Stage 1 is designed to help improve cardiorespiratory fitness levels in apparently healthy sedentary clients using a target intensity below ventilatory threshold 1 (VT1) and involves steady-state aerobic exercise.

A **stage 2** workout consists of a mix of recovery intervals just below VT1 (moderate intensity) and work intervals performed at an intensity just above VT1 (challenging to hard intensity). Once clients become accustomed to stage 2 intervals and have shown positive signs of adapting to the physical demands, they can begin performing moderately intense steady-state cardio exercise just above VT1, if desired.

A **stage 3** workout includes the client moving in and out of training zones 1, 2, and 3.

A **stage 4** workout involves interval training integrating all four training zones.

Stage 5 focuses on drills that help improve conditioning using linear, multidirectional, and sport-specific activities performed as conditioning and often combines high-intensity interval training with small-sided games and agility drills. Common postural deviations that clients may exhibit while engaging in cardiorespiratory training include round shoulders and forward head, an anterior pelvic tilt, or adducted and internally rotated knees and pronated feet.

Caution should be made to monitor a client's posture during cardiorespiratory exercise.

Core Training Concepts

Core training is critical for improving posture, enhancing performance, increasing injury resistance, and accelerating injury rehabilitation. The core is defined by the structures that make up the lumbopelvic-hip complex (LPHC) and includes the global and local core musculature. Local core muscles generally attach on or near the vertebrae. Local muscles provide dynamic control of the spinal segments, limiting excessive compression, shear, and rotational forces between spinal segments.

Global core muscles are more superficial on the trunk. Global muscles act to move the trunk, transfer loads between the upper and lower extremities, and stabilize the spine by stabilizing multiple segments together as functional units. When designing a core training program, the local and global muscles should both be trained to develop proper core stability and overall movement efficiency.

Core strength is imperative for maintaining the spine's natural curvatures, both at rest and during movement. Large curvatures of the spine away from the midline are considered abnormal and may be
considered either structural or functional scoliosis. Core training has been demonstrated to improve injury resistance by contributing to more coordinated motion between the trunk and lower extremities during high-energy, sport-specific activities. When developing a core training program, emphasize increasing proprioceptive demand initially instead of increasing the external resistance. Additionally, emphasize the quality of movement across the LPHC.

Many variables can be manipulated when designing a core training program, including planes of motion, ranges of motion, speed of motion, volume, and exercise modalities. Be cautious not to change too many variables at one time when progressing an exercise program to make sure that the client can demonstrate appropriate mastery at each stage.

Initially, start with core exercises that involve little motion of the spine and target the local core musculature. Example exercises consist of (but are not limited to) marching, floor/ball bridge, floor/ball cobra, plank, side plank, dead bug, and Palloff press. The next-level core exercise progression incorporates more motion at the spine that also targets global core muscles. Example exercises can be seen in the following (but are not limited to) floor/ball crunch, back extension, reverse crunch, knee-up, and cable rotation, lift, and chop.

The last core exercise progression involves explosive movement through the trunk and extremities. Example exercises encompass (but are not limited to) medicine ball chest pass, ball medicine ball pullover throw, front medicine ball oblique throw, side medicine ball oblique throw, medicine ball soccer throw, medicine ball wood chop throw, and medicine ball overhead throw.

Balance Training Concepts

Balance training is a critical component of an exercise program to optimize performance, improve injury resistance, and enhance injury rehabilitation. Maintaining balance involves the ability of an individual to control the position of the center of gravity over the base of support.

Types of balance include static (stationary body position), semi-dynamic (the base supporting the body is in movement), and dynamic (ever-changing base of support) and can be manipulated to change the level of difficulty during a balance training program.

The balance mechanism involves three key senses:
- Vision, which is typically used to provide information to the central nervous system about the body's location in space.
- The vestibular senses, which are controlled by sensory receptors in the inner ear and provide the brain information about spatial orientation and the movement of the head in space.
- Somatosensation, which is the ability to feel changes in pressure on the skin, muscle length, and joint angles.

Balance training has been evidenced to improve performance and reduce injury rates in athletes when incorporated into a comprehensive injury prevention program that is carried throughout the course of an athletic season. Strong evidence demonstrates that balance training programs can reduce the risk of falls in healthy older adults.

Fitness professionals should always emphasize safety when designing a progressive balance training program, especially for clients with a history of injuries or a current injury. When developing a balance training program, emphasize a safe and progressive increase in proprioceptive demand based on the client's performance. Many variables can be manipulated when designing a balance training program, including planes, range, and speed of motion, as well as the proprioceptive environment. Be cautious not to change too many variables at one time when progressing an exercise program to make sure that the client can demonstrate appropriate mastery at each stage.

Plyometric (Reactive) Training Concepts

Plyometric training, also known as jump or reactive training, is a form of exercise that uses explosive movements, such as bounding, jumping, or powerful upper body movements, to develop muscular power. Employing plyometric training develops efficient control and production of ground reaction forces, which can be used to protect the body from harm with a greater speed of movement.

Clients must possess adequate core strength, joint stability, and range of motion and must balance efficiently prior to performing explosive plyometric exercises. The integrated performance paradigm posits that to move with precision, forces have to be loaded (eccentrically), stabilized (isometrically), and then unloaded or accelerated (concentrically). The three distinct phases of the stretch-shortening cycle involved in a plyometric exercise include the eccentric or loading phase, the amortization phase or transition phase, and the concentric or unloading phase.

Plyometric exercises increase the rate of force production (power) and motor unit recruitment. Plyometric exercises should progress from simple to intermediate to advanced movements and from low intensity to moderate intensity to high intensity. Intensity should be prescribed by the client's ability to execute the movement and maintain adequate training technique. If technique is lost, the intensity should drop until proper technique is achieved. Plyometric intensity describes the amount of effort or stress applied by the muscles, connective tissue, and joints during plyometric drills and by the distance covered (height of a jump).

Plyometric volume is defined as the number of foot contacts, throws, or catches. An example would be the completion of three sets of five squat jumps, equating to a volume of 15.

A general recommendation is to allow at least 1 day between intense plyometric training sessions. At least 48 to 72 hours between sessions are the recommended

guidelines when implementing plyometrics for novice individuals. Since plyometric training involves jumping, bounding, and other explosive movements, it is essential to teach proper landing and rebounding mechanics. As a general rule, recovery times of 60 to 120 seconds between drills should be sufficient for full recovery, but this is dictated by the client's fitness level. When introducing plyometric exercises—especially to new or beginner clients—the movements should initially involve small jumps, and clients should hold the landing position for 3–5 seconds and make any adjustments necessary to correct faulty postures
before performing the next jump.

The next progression is to involve jumps with more amplitude and dynamic motion performed with a repetitive tempo. The last progression includes exercises that are performed as fast and as explosively as
possible.

Speed, Agility, and Quickness (SAQ) Training Concepts

SAQ training is an effective and appropriate method of fitness training stimulating muscular, neurological, connective tissue, and even cardiovascular fitness adaptations. SAQ exercises can promote improvements in physical performance and sustain youthful movement throughout life.

SAQ training will allow clients to enhance their ability to accelerate, decelerate, and dynamically stabilize their entire body during high-velocity movements in all planes of motion. Speed, the product of stride rate and stride length, refers to the velocity of distance covered divided by time. Agility necessitates the ability to start (or accelerate), stop (or decelerate and stabilize), and change direction while maintaining postural control.

Quickness is the ability to respond to a stimulus and appropriately change the motion of the body in response to that stimulus. Stride rate refers to the number of strides taken in a given amount of time (or distance). The distance covered in one stride is referred to as the Stride length. Proper running mechanics will enable the client to maximize force generation through biomechanical efficiency. Components of an SAQ program can significantly improve the physical health profile of apparently healthy, sedentary, nonathletic adults and those with medical or health limitations.

SAQ programs for youth have been found to decrease the likelihood of athletic injury, increase the likelihood of exercise participation later in life, and improve physical fitness. SAQ training for older adults may help prevent age-related decreases in bone density, coordinative ability, and muscular power. The high-intensity, short bouts of SAQ drills make them a valid choice for interval training protocols with appropriate nonathletic populations, including weight-loss clients.

Resistance Training Concepts

The GAS model outlines three stages of response to stress: alarm reaction, resistance development, and exhaustion. The alarm reaction stage, the initial reaction to a stressor, can include fatigue, joint stiffness, or delayed onset muscle soreness. The resistance development stage involves numerous physiological changes that ultimately lead to training adaptations that promote increases in performance. Prolonged or intolerable amounts of stress lead to the exhaustion stage, which is characterized by stress fractures, muscle strains and ligament sprains, joint pain, and emotional fatigue.

The principle of specificity often referred to as the SAID principle, describes the body's responses and adaptations to exercise. Mechanical specificity is the weight and movements placed upon the body. Neuromuscular specificity refers to the speed of contraction and exercise selection. Metabolic specificity refers to the energy demand placed on the body. The main adaptations that occur from resistance training include stabilization, muscular endurance, hypertrophy, strength, and power.

Stabilization is the body's ability to provide optimal dynamic joint support to maintain correct posture during all movements. Muscular endurance is the ability to produce and maintain force production for
prolonged periods of time. Muscular hypertrophy is the enlargement of skeletal muscle fibers. Strength is the ability of the neuromuscular system to produce internal tension, specifically in the muscles and connective tissues that tug on the bones, to overwhelm an external force.

Power is the capacity of the neuromuscular system to produce the greatest possible force in the shortest possible time. Acute variables include repetitions, sets, training intensity, repetition tempo, rest intervals, training volume, training frequency, training duration, exercise selection, and exercise order. There are numerous training systems that can be used to structure resistance training programs for a variety of effects. Several of the most common training systems include warm-up set, single set, multiple set, pyramid, superset, complex training, drop set, giant set, rest-pause set, circuit training, peripheral heart action, split routine, vertical loading, and horizontal loading.

Fitness professionals must safeguard their clients from harm. This requires maintaining a safe environment, ensuring proper equipment set up, using appropriate spotting procedures, and monitoring exercise techniques using the five kinetic chain checkpoints. Resistance exercises should initially focus on optimizing ideal movement patterns. Once a client displays adequate movement competency, resistance exercises should progress in a systematic fashion using three steps:

(1) stabilization-focused exercises
(2) strength-focused exercises, and
(3) power-focused exercises.

Understanding the Corrective Exercise Continuum (CEX) of the NASM

The aim of Corrective Exercises are to help people move and feel better, whether it's while exercising or just going through everyday life. To accomplish this, it needs a true and in-depth understanding of four phases that comprise the Corrective Exercise Continuum (CEx). These phases are:

- Inhibit
- Lengthen
- Activate
- Integrate

Corrective Exercises are techniques used by health & fitness professionals to address and correct movement compensations and imbalances. Personal trainers, massage therapists and chiropractors, commonly use these exercises to aid their clients move and feel better both during a workout session and through each day.

Within these conditions, the [NASM Corrective Exercise Specialization](#) educates you on how to use an array of dynamic and static assessments to identify imbalances and use the results to fashion out efficient plans for your clients using NASM's world-renowned Corrective Exercise Continuum.

NASM'S 4-Step of Corrective Exercise Continuum (CEX)

The Corrective Exercise Continuum (CEx) is an easy to understand yet highly effective four-step process used by fitness professionals with their clients and athletes to help them improve, and ultimately, rectify common movement compensations.

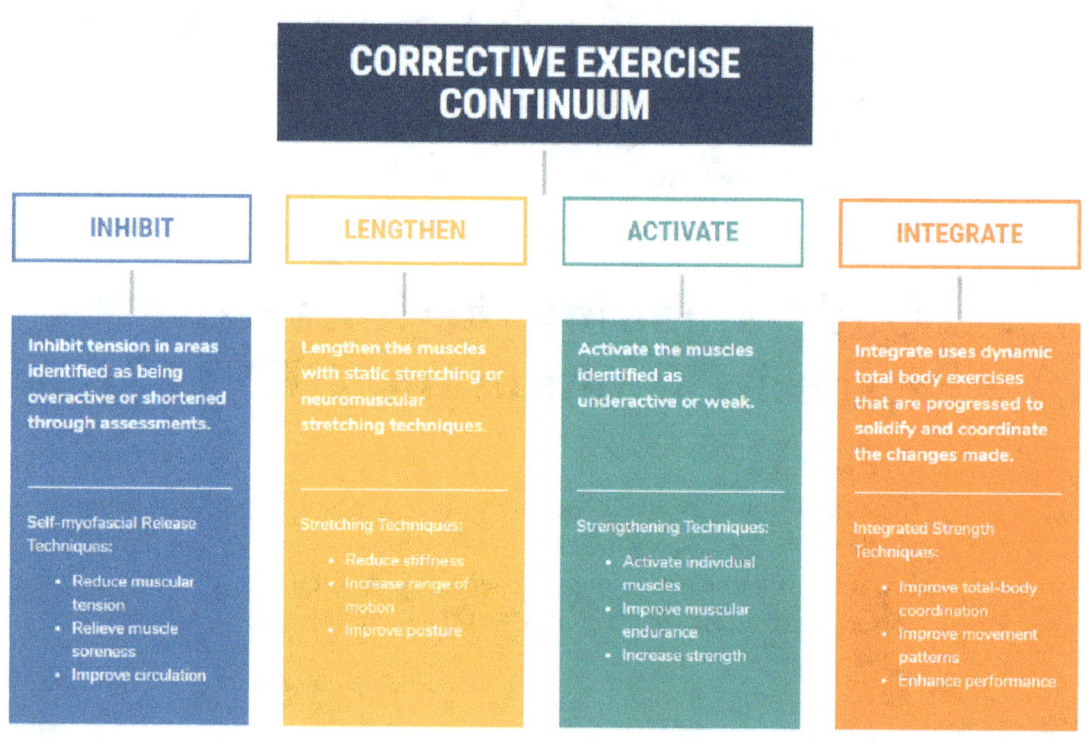

Here we have a breakdown of the four steps and how best to maximize them:

CEX PHASE 1: Inhibit Overactive Muscles

Inhibit is the number one phase in the Corrective Exercise Continuum. The end result of the Inhibit phase is to reduce or control the activity of the nervous system that innervates the myofascial. It is vital to recognize that muscles known as overactive (via the movement assessments) should receive inhibition techniques.

There are numerous corrective exercises to suppress **overactive** muscles, such as percussion devices, foam rolling, or hands-on techniques like massage and instrument-assisted soft-tissue manipulation. However, a good number of these techniques need additional licensure. It stands then that foam rolling is the most common for the Corrective Exercise Specialist.

The foam roller is presumed to work via two primary mechanisms:

1) it affects local tissue dysfunction
2) it influences the autonomic nervous system

The ultimate aim of foam rolling is to ready the muscle for phase 2, Lengthening, by working on local tissue mechanics and making the muscle more susceptible to stretching via afferent central nervous system (CNS) pathways.

Research submits that foam rolling before stretching leads to enhanced improvements in flexibility and joint range of motion.

CEX PHASE 2: Stretch Shortened Muscles

Lengthening is the second phase in the Corrective Exercise Continuum. As opposed to popular belief, muscle fibers are not *stretch*ed out by stretching. Lengthening can be seen as the elongation of mechanically shortened muscles and connective tissue via a nervous system response. In this process, there is a decrease in muscle spindle activity and motor neuron excitability
.

An essential aspect of static stretching that all professionals need to understand is that the more the muscle and connective tissue be
gin to encounter force, the easier it is to elongate, which in turn allows for improved range motion.

Stretching has mechanical effects such as increasing muscle compliance, but the real advantage of stretching is a *"psycho-physiological"* effect, the increased stretch tolerance.

In simpler terms, static stretching will *"calm a muscle down,"* which allows for improved length-tension relationships, force-couple relationships, improvement in range of motion,and enhanced movement patterns.

A common mistake made by most people is to stretch those muscles which feel "tight." Lengthening should only be used on those muscles which have been identified as short and overactive. However, because of the response of certain stretch receptors, muscles that are long are more often described as feeling strung up than those that are short. It is, therefore, imperative that the findings of the movement assessments are used to direct the corrective exercises to integrate into your programming.

It may help to consider Phases 1 and 2 of the Corrective Exercise Continuum as the *Mo*vement parts of corrective exercises. Inhibition and Lengthening are both used before activation to work on tissue extensibility and joint range of motion before isolated strengthening. Muscle functioning properly is dependent on proper movement of the joints.

CEX PHASE 3: Activate Underactive Muscles

The third phase on the list of Corrective Exercise Continuum is the Activation of the underactive muscles. Activation is the stimulation of underactive/lengthened myofascial tissue. Amongst the activation methods available, NASM proposes the usage of isolated strengthening for Corrective Exercise Specialists.

Isolated strengthening is the grouping of corrective exercises used to *isolate* particular muscles, and in some cases, to focus on a particular part of a specific muscle, to increase intramuscular coordination, and to improve force production capabilities. Intramuscular coordination is said to have been achieved when a muscle has the optimal firing rate, motor unit synchronization, and the optimal motor unit activation.

Similar to an intrastate highway, isolated strengthening focuses on one muscle and is unconcerned with crossing over *state* lines into alien muscles. Thus, there is a need for accuracy as these corrective exercises have to be carried out in controlled environments. To focus on a specific muscle, stability and support, the fitness professional is urged to use the necessary tools and equipment.

An example could also be activation of the gluteus for a client that demonstrates knee valgus, indicating an underactive gluteus. The gluteus is a primary hip abductor but has anterior fibers that also produce hip flexion and medial rotation – while, on the other hand, posterior fibers produce hip extension and lateral rotation.

The client demonstrated flexion compensation and medial hip rotation. Thus, the CEx Specialist must highlight the posterior fibers. To achieve this, the CEx Specialist may have the individual also produce slight hip extension during a hip abduction exercise, this will activate the posterior fibers and middle fibres. Further, considering this, underactive core muscles also are related to knee valgus. The client needs to maintain a stable spine while engaged in the medius activation exercise, as a result, professionals fitness coaches need to pick the right positions for this workout.

The side-lying hip abduction exercise is one that strengthens the gluteus medius, the CEx Specialists can aid the individual in performing this exercise, pressing the working leg back into a wall, known as the wall slide. The client can then maintain a neutral spine in this position. Specific fibres are targeted within a particular muscle to reduce the knee valgus compensation.

Fitness professionals are always encouraged to get the individuals into optimal positions for these kinds of exercises. To this end, fitness professionals are encouraged to use tools and equipment.

This sort of training isn't permanent, and the stronger the client gets, the less he has to rely on his training wheels.

CEX PHASE 4: Integrate With Multi-Joint Movements

The final phase of the Corrective Exercise Continuum, Integration, is when actions are taken on steps 1-3.

Functional movement patterns can be retaught through Integration techniques. This is done by reestablishing neuromuscular control and promoting coordinated movement. Intermuscular coordination is well aided by integration exercises. The various exercises function separately and they do not disturb their separate functions.

It is important that integration exercises are very functional such that the movement is important and engaged on a daily basis. The exercises should start out with focused and slow movements done in a defined setting. This should be done in a defined setting such that the client can maintain an optimal form.

Integration exercises should include simple tasks that the individual would carry out on their day-to-day routines. The exercises should take place in a controlled environment with simple and easy-to-do tasks to help the client adapt faster.' With time, the level of difficulty in the exercise would also increase, focused exercise should also be included. Phase 1 of the OPT model resistance training often looks like the integration exercises.

An example of an Integrated exercise for the client with knee valgus may be a ball-wall squat with a mini-band around the knees. The squat pattern is functional, and the mini band will encourage the client to maintain proper knee position during the movement. As the client improves, the mini band may be removed (thus removing the feedback), and weights may be added to increase the resistance.

This could eventually be progressed by squatting without the use of a ball and then to changing base of support by performing a split squat or lunge. The lunge may be progressed through the three cardinal planes of motion, and finally, a squat jump may be added to enhance the eccentric demand.

Focusing on the eccentric portion of all Integration exercises and improving postural control in all planes of motion may help to reduce specific injuries.

Like the Activation phase, optimal form is vital during the Integration exercises.

Practice Questions

- **Reciprocal inhibition is:**

A. Response to stimuli that activates movement in muscles

B. Muscle groups produce movement around a joint by moving at the same time

C. When a muscle allows another muscle to contract by relaxing

D. The resting length of a muscle and the tension that the muscle is able to produce at that resting length

Answer:

The Correct Answer is 'C'. When a muscle allows another muscle to contract by relaxing

C perfectly defines what reciprocal inhibition is. The muscle relaxes, meaning it is inhibited, to allow its opposite to contract, meaning it reciprocates.

2. What is Relative flexibility?

A. The range of motion joint moves in without pain

B. The neuromuscular system allowing agonists, antagonists, and stabilizers to synergistically produce muscle forces

C. An increase in the normal movement and functionality of a joint, this alters the range of motion
D. The human movement system finds the movement path that has the least resistance

Answer:

The Correct Answer is D. The human movement system finds the movement path that has the least resistance

Relative flexibility handles the ROM within a normal comfortable level of mobility, i.e. the least resistive. This is as opposed to maximal flexibility, which handles the ROM limits about joints.

3. What kind of relationship does overactivity and tightness within a muscle tend to have ?
A. A relative relationship
B. A direct relationship
C. There is no relationship
D. An inverse relationship

Answer:

The Correct Answer is B. A direct relationship

Overactivity has been shown to lead to tightness. As muscle becomes more active, especially when hypertrophy is experienced, this leads to a gradual decline in mobility and ROM.

4. What type of flexibility is static stretching considered?
A. Active flexibility
B. Functional flexibility
C. Immobile flexibility
D. Corrective flexibility

Answer:

The Correct Answer is D. Corrective flexibility

Static flexibility helps improve range of motion and reduce tightness, both of which are considered deficiencies or a cause for imbalance requiring correction.

5. What is Autogenic inhibition?
A. A process in which proper muscle contraction is inhibited by excessive tightness of the muscle, this could lead to injury
B. A process in which tension impulses are greater than contraction impulses, leading to relaxation of the muscle
C. A process in which neural impulses recruit muscles in order to produce force using mechanoreceptors
D. A process where inhibitory action to muscle fibers will lead to excessive increases in muscle length

Answer:

The Correct Answer is B. A process in which tension impulses are greater than contraction impulses, leading to relaxation of the muscle

An autogenic action is one that responds to natural circumstances which is the case where tension is greater than contraction, leading to inhibition.

6. What muscles need to be statically stretched?
A. All the muscles of the lower body
B. Muscles that have been identified as overactive
C. The major muscles at each kinetic chain checkpoint
D. Muscles that have been identified as weak

Answer:

The Correct Answer is B. Muscles that have been identified as overactive

This is because overactive muscles tend to tighten and shorten over time, so in order to correct and counteract this issue, static stretching should be employed.

7. Why is myofascial release beneficial before a workout?

A. It can help flush out excess lactic acid
B. It can break up fascial adhesions
C. It can be used as a method of muscle activation
D. It can prevent muscle soreness

Answer:

The Correct Answer is B. It can break up fascial adhesions

Because the myofascial release is a superficial release, meaning it doesn't target the deeper muscle layers, it is a safe way to promote pre-workout readiness. By breaking up fascial adhesions, you can promote better mobility, ROM and in turn, force production while reducing injury risk.

8. What type of stretching needs to be avoided if postural distortions are present?
A. Self-myofascial release (SMR)
B. Ballistic stretching
C. Active-isolated stretching
D. Static stretching

Answer:

The Correct Answer is B. Active-isolated stretching

Active-isolated stretching is designated for improving ROM in limbs about a single joint axis through the use of reciprocal inhibition. This also poses potential risks when active-isolated stretching is employed along the spinal column.

9. Which of these is pattern overload?
A. Walking every day for 20 minutes
B. Extended periods of sitting every day
C. Variety of core strength exercises at every training session
D. Superset resistance training several days per week

Answer:

The Correct Answer is B. Extended periods of sitting every day.

Pattern overload occurs when a habit or movement pattern is engaged regularly for hours on end. For office workers and those with a sedentary lifestyle, sitting certainly promotes pattern overload which leads to poor hip mobility amongst other things.

10. Which ligament receives high stress during the inverted hurdler's stretch?
A. Posterior cruciate ligament
B. Anterior cruciate ligament
C. Medial collateral ligament
D. Lateral collateral ligament

Answer:

The Correct Answer is C. Medial collateral ligament

The MCL is greatly strained during an inverted hurdle stretch as compared to the other knee ligaments due to the position.

Chapter 6

Professional Development and Responsibility

This part evaluates the candidate's knowledge of business basics, marketing practices, sales methods, business development, equipment maintenance, professional limitations of the CPT, proper emergency situation procedures, CPT occupational limitations, retaining professional credentials, use of credible health and fitness educational resources, professional growth opportunities, ethical standards, and professional codes of conduct.

Health and Fitness in Modern Times

NASM's methodologies and fitness work efficiently for any fitness goal-oriented client because of its focus on scientific principles. NASM suggests that all fitness professionals maintain a focus on an evidence-based practice attaining the highest levels of success.

Evidence-based practice is the conscientious use of current best evidence in making decisions about the clients' welfare. With NASM's revolutionary approach to physical exercise, they designed an OPT model that is backed with ample evidence as to how it works. Medical conditions that occur instantly but can be diagnosed and treated in no time are acute diseases. While a chronic illness is one which remains persistently, or probably never gets cured. Overweight and obesity are terms for a bodyweight heavier than the average or expected weight for a healthy person of a particular height. Obesity is usually because of exess fat.

An overweight or obese person is more likely to be chronically ill. Cardiovascular illness is a broad description for multiple chronic illnesses of the blood vessels and heart, such as cardiac arrest, heart attacks, stroke, arrhythmia, and heart valve problems.

Hypertension is one major risk factor for cardiac diseases and stroke, which are the leading causes of death worldwide. Cholesterol, a proteinous and fatty acid-containing substance, is a waxy solid found in the blood. Diabetes is a disease of the blood glucose being at an elevated level. Glucose comes from food. A hormone, insulin, is secreted from the pancreas and it breaks down glucose for it to be used as energy for activities.

Cancer is a rapid, abnormal growth of cells which is linked to several genetic and environmental causes. COPD is a general term for lung infections. They are marked by symptoms such as breath loss, airflow restriction, and accelerated decline of lung function.

Two issues are most frequent at the foot and ankle, and these are plantar fasciitis and ankle sprains. Sprains happen when a person's ankle gets twisted, or rolled out of joint, causing the ligaments to tear. Plantar fasciitis, on the other hand, causes pain in the plantar fascia tissue located under the feet.

The LPHC comprises the lower back, pelvis, hip musculoskeletal and abdominal structures. This region is known as the "core." The LPHC is a vital structure in the human body because it links the upper and lower halves of a person. Dysfunction of the shoulder is rampant in the general population, most commonly in people who lift weights overhead regularly.

Frequent physical activity has time and time again been proven to amend several chronic and musculoskeletal diseases. Understanding the methods of practice for all adjacent allied health professionals, as well as the required local laws and regulations, will make sure CPTs are working within their scope of practice at all times. Networking with other allied health practitioners and certified fitness professionals and colleagues can lead to great levels of success in the fitness industry.

A NASM-CPT is required to be conversant with **the NASM Code of Professional Conduct,** and adhere to it.

NASM CPT CODE OF ETHICS

NASM has a code of conduct set for public and professional protection. All candidates and Certified Professionals are expected to act in line with the Code of Professional Conduct, which is stated below.

Being Professional

Each NASM Certified Professional must give top-notch professional services and client care in their practice. They should:
- Obey the NASM Code of Professional Conduct fully and behave respectfully ; Conduct themselves in a manner that merits the respect from the public, their colleagues and the NASM body.
- Treat every client and colleague and client with utter respect.
- Refrain from making derogatory or untrue assumptions concerning the practices of their colleagues and patrons.
- Communicate with propriety and professionalism at all times, in all written, spoken and non-verbal activities.

5. Maintain a safe environment for clients at all times. This requires the Certified Professional to:

a. Refrain from diagnosing or treating injuries except for basic first aid purposes, or in the case that the Certified Professional has a legal license to offer that treatment at that time.

b. Not train any clients with a diagnosed health condition unless the Certified Professional is adequately trained to do so, follows procedures prescribed and supervised by a licensed medical professional, or if the Certified Professional has a legal license to do so at the time.

c. Not provide training to a client prior to receiving and reviewing a current health-history questionnaire signed by the client.

d. Always hold a current CPR (cardiopulmonary resuscitation) and AED (automated external defibrillator) certification from a NASM-approved provider.

6. Refer the client immediately to the appropriate medical practitioner as soon as, the Certified Professional:

a. Notices any change in the client's health status or medication;

b. Is aware of any undiagnosed illness, injury, or risk factor; or an administered suspension or withdrawal of credentials (Disciplinary Action) section 31;

c. Becomes aware of unusual pain and/or discomfort experienced by the client in the course of the training session, which warrants professional care, in which case the Certified Professional must end the session instantly.

7. Recommend other healthcare professionals to the client, when nutritional and supplemental advice is requested, except if the Certified Professional has been specifically trained or is certified to do so, at that time.

8. Maintain proper personal hygiene as is suitable for a health and fitness environment.

9. Wear clean, professional and decent clothing.

10. Maintain current certification status and reputation by obtaining all necessary requirements for continued education.

Be Confidential

A Certified Professional must regard the confidential information of all clients at all times, and:

1. Protect the client's confidentiality in all advertisements, discussions and every other way, unless with the written permission of the client, or when legally required, or in the advent of medical requirements.
2. Protect the clients' interests when clients are legally minors, or incapacitated to willingly grant consent without the legal permission of ta guardian or suitable third party.
3. Keep and discard of client records by security-conscious means.

Act Legally and Ethically

Each Certified Professional must abide by every legal requirement within the required jurisdiction. In his/her official role, every Certified Professional should:

1. Obey every local, state, federal, and provincial laws, rules, and professional guidelines.
2. Accept full responsibility for each of his/her actions.
3. Maintain accurate and honest records.
4. Uphold all existing copyright, intellectual property rights, and trademark regulations.

NASM may revoke or the certification of an offending individual who is or has been convicted of, plead guilty to, or plead no contest to a felony or misdemeanor or has been found to have been negligent or legally responsible for the injury or harm of an in performing in his or her professional capacity or have misrepresented his/her qualifications to provide services, including opinions or advice, to the public.

Business Practice.

Each Certified Professional must be honest, integrous, and lawful. In performing his or her duty, the Certified Professional must:

1. Maintain adequate liability insurance;
2. Maintain truthful and substantial progress notes for every of his/her clients;
3.. Accurately inform the public of the kind of services rendered as well as their qualification to offer these stated services;
4. Truthfully represent all their professional certifications and qualifications;
5. Put up advertisement in an honest manner that fully represents their services, without using harmful or provocative language and visuals;
6. Maintain accurate financial, contract, appointment, and tax records including original receipts of at least four years; and
7. Keep all the local, state, federal, and providence laws and employer rules regarding harassment and discrimination, including sexual harassment.

Professional Personal Training

From working in a large fitness club, to training clients in the comfort of their residences, fitness professionals have numerous options to build a personal training practice with a consistent patronage of clients. An alternate employment route that fitness professionals tend to take is starting up a fitness business that could include working with clients in their homes, running outdoor group workout programs, or opening a studio.

With evolving technological innovations, numerous opportunities are now available for offering fitness training online. Working independently allows a fitness professional to determine his or her own income rates and earn as much as he or she desires, if they are well qualified. However all taxes, insurance and operational costs, have to be accounted for.

A move towards success as a CPT is to provide competent customer service. To sell personal training services is to ask a client to commit to a fitness regimen that will better his or her life - fitness wise. It is a solution offered to solving their fitness and health problems, and if the communication channel with a prospective client is well-created, sales will feel natural and automatic.

Forecasting is a technique that can determine the number of customers that need to be serviced, in order to reach a preferred financial goal per year. Marketing is an important process of passing across the needs that a specific product or service will meet for a potential client. The Four Ps of marketing are price, promotion, product and place. Social media and other digital marketing strategies are extremely vital for establishing a fitness business in the modern day.

Continuing education courses are not only important to gain recertification; they can teach fitness professionals how to work with niche populations, thus granting them the ability to expand their fitness business to new and exciting areas. The most common methods of earning CEUs are attending seminars or workshops, or completing online educational courses. Also, CEUs can be obtained by participating in livestream webinars, reading fitness and health articles and passing a quiz or test, or making contributions to the industry by creating content for fitness education programs, speaking at seminars, and presenting webinars.

Practice Questions

- **Which is a niche in the training business?**

A. Private gym teaching
B. Women's fitness
C. Independent contracting
D. Small group training
Answer:
The Correct Answer is B. Women's fitness

Most fitness niches are often identified by a specific theme. This theme can be specified by population, demographic, or a method of training. According to the question, only 'B' fits this description. This is because women fitness is a designated population group for training. The other options only describe other business models in the personal training industry. They are not examples of a niche.

- **What additional certification is a NASM PT required to have?**

A. NCCA
B. CPR
C. First Aid
D. Undergraduate degree
Answer:

The Correct Answer is B. CPR

Other than the essential high school diploma or any other certification that is equivalent, to become a certified personal trainer, you are also required to produce a currently active CPR/AED certification.

3. Which of the following is ideal when communicating with a possible new client that is improperly performing a fitness exercise?
A. Tell them that you know the proper way to do the exercise
B. Offering them a better way of performing the exercise
C. Informing them about the benefits of the exercise
D. Asking if you can suggest something

Answer:
The Correct Answer is A. Tell them that you know the proper way to do the exercise.

When trying to convince a client, you should start with the benefits of doing the exercise right. This way, you are able to prevent further defensive resistance or wrong performance that the client have.

More importantly, it also allows them to feel instructed rather than feel judged or insulted. It all begins with you being able to validate their attempts and then follow up with a correction that is wrapped in a suggestive manner rather than as a command. You can maintain great communication and rapport without psychological resistance and a bruised ego.

4. Which one of these is a part of in-house personal training?
A. The trainer pays a health club so as to train clients
B. The trainer is paid an hourly income with benefits
C. The trainer is required to travel and use portable equipment
D. The trainer owns a facility and bears responsibility for its running and ordinances

Answer:
The Correct Answer is C. The trainer is required to travel and use portable equipment

Being an in-house personal trainer means that the trainer is open to house calls requiring them to train clients right in their homes. In order to acheive maximum efficiency and effectiveness, it is highly recommended that you make use of portable equipment that can be carried around easily. Instruments such as resistance bands and suspension trainers are advised.

5. How should a trainer reach out to their client after collecting their contact information?
A. Call the potential client no earlier than 2 to 3 days after
B. Approach the client at their subsequent presence at the gym
C. Mail a handwritten card within the first 24 hours
D. Email the client after a few days of meeting with them
Answer:
The Correct Answer is 'C'. Mail a handwritten card within the first 24 hours

It is commonplace to put a phone call through or send an email. However, when you send a handwritten card by mail, it is mostly considered by most people as considerate, personal and classy. This can boost the impression you leave on your client immediately. It shows that you are a personal trainer that care and is committed. This way, the client can expect so much more from you.

6. When is a trainer required to give a percentage of their session fees?
A. When employed and working full-time at a commercial fitness club
B. Working at a commercial fitness club as an independent contractor
C. As the owner of a facility
D. When offering in-home personal training services
Answer:
The Correct Answer is 'B'. Working at a commercial fitness club as an independent contractor.

In a set up where the personal trainer makes use of an existing 3rd part commercial gym for his or her business, they would be expected and required to pay off a percentage of their total earnings and session fee as a form of compensation for using their equipment.

7. Which of these is an aspect of independent contractor work as a personal trainer?
A. Although the trainer is required to transport equipment, there aren't any overhead costs.

B. A trainer with multiple fitness certifications have a chance of getting paid more
C. The trainer is only required to work an as-needed basis
D. The trainer has the liberty to market or even target a specific population

Answer:

The Correct Answer is C. The trainer works on an as-needed basis

Because an independent trainer is not bound to any employment conditions, quotas, or a roster, they can work at will, as booked and needed by clients. While D and A and B may apply to an independent contractor, they are not exclusive to that business model.

8. Out of the following options, which one of them is a good reason to stay within your scope of practice?
A. To become a high-quality trainer
B. To avoid injury and liability
C. To ensure a long career
D. To maintain the reputation of the gym

Answer:

The Correct Answer is B. To avoid injury and liability

A personal trainer's scope of practice sits within the initial assessment of goals and readiness for exercise, designing of the exercise programs, and safe, effective instruction of exercises in the program. Anything beyond that could lead to injury and liability since a PT is not qualified or licensed to diagnose or treat any conditions.

9. Why is the uncompromising of your customer service such an essential part of being a personal trainer?
A. It is necessary for the personal trainer to be considered ethical
B. It provides an exceptionally valuable experience to the client
C. It is necessary to develop your reputation as a decent trainer
D. It shows that you are unwilling to compromise on your personal beliefs

Answer:

The Correct Answer is B. It provides an exceptionally valuable experience to the client

The fitness industry is quite saturated, so in order to have a shot at standing out, providing a second to none experience is a basic consideration. While A and C are essential to being a good PT, they don't impact a client's impression of you in an immediate and direct way.

10. Which is a suitable pricing strategy for training?
A. A price higher than what is comfortable for the clients
B. On par with prices in other similar areas
C. On par with your competition
D. More than your competition
Answer:
The Correct Answer is C. On par with your competition

When pricing your services as a trainer, you don't want to underprice. This will lead you to earn less than you potentially could and devalues your brand in the long run. Overpricing your services, unless they are extremely niched down, won't gain you much traction since there are other similar services more competitively priced.

Chapter 7

Client Relations and Behavioral Coaching

In the Client Relations and Behavioral Coaching aspect of the NASM CPT, exams include:

- Topics like client-CPT professional relationships.
- Teaching clients about lifestyle changes.
- Client communication.
- Active listening.
- Obstacles to behavior change.
- SMART goal development.
- Psychological responses to exercise.

This encompasses a concept most refer to as "change psychology." Reason being that the main aim of a health coach is to inspire a change of habits and behaviours from unhealthy ones, to those that result in positive outcomes. This is achieved through effective communication, and is why questions from this domain will test one mainly on the quality of communication as a profession trainer.

Topics in this domain include the best practices for listening, which are: active listening, listening to offer support, and also the quality and nature of feedback. The exam will also assess your ability to identify barriers to success towards client goals.

However, this domain holds the lowest weighting, so you should attach less focus to it. Having said that, we must mention that this domain is essential for personal research and education, especially because it covers the business and entrepreneurial fundamentals of all personal training.

Essentially, as a qualified professional trainer, you are a business person who runs a business. But let us go back to the exam. It is a brief assessment of the topic, and only really examines you on some broad stroke basics of making income as a professional trainer. The four P's of marketing - product, price, place, and promotion - as well as effective sales strategies are the core components of this aspect.

A Psychological View on Exercise

Psychology is an important component to human habit change and plays a key role in adopting exercise as a regular habit.

Intrinsic motivation describes the desire to do something that comes from within an individual; it is required for long-term habit development. Motivation to exercise differs from one individual to another and will change over time, thus motives should be reevaluated over time. Most factors that serve as barriers to exercise are often lack of time, unrealistic goals, lack of social support, social physique anxiety, inconvenience, and being double-minded, but all barriers can be either reduced or dissolved with some basic, realistic suggestions.

Lack of time is solved by proper time management and resetting of priorities. Goals that are not feasible become a barrier to exercise, thus, the fitness professional should help clients to plan the outcome and processes of their goals. Sometimes, people feel anxious about how others perceive their bodies and it it can be a hindrance to doing exercise. Providing clients with activities that reduce this type of anxiety will create a comfortable exercise environment for them. Seeing exercise as inconvenient can be overcome by making the exercise experience as exciting as possible, by providing customer service in clean, well-kept facilities and also providing clients options to exercise outside the walls of a commercial fitness establishment.

Ambivalence or being double-minded to exercise happens when a person has mixed feelings about exercise and sees the merits and disadvantages to participation. Social influences about exercise can come from other people, the internet, or the

environment; these influences both direct people towards and away from exercise. Social support consists of a source that provides, and a type of support (instrumental, emotional, informational, and companionship)' Clients will have different needs and expectations of social support.

Another form of support is the instrumental type. It involves the obvious, physical aids that assist people with the ability to exercise. For instance, providing transportation to a fitness facility, assisting with childcare, or packing a person's gym bag for them. Emotional support comes from being concerned and empathising with someone's experience with exercise. Being empathetic involves the ability to relate to the way another person feels or views about a situation. One major reason why a client will seek out a fitness professional is informational support. It includes providing accurate and relevant information about exercise and fitness.

Companionship support is when somebody exercises with another person. Group influences on exercise are the impressions held by other people over whether or not a person exercises and can come from family members, parents, exercise leaders, exercise groups, or the surrounding community. A parent's influence can impact children and adolescents, whereas instrumental support is often recognised as a highly influential form of support. The exercise leader sets the atmosphere for the class and is responsible for creating an inviting and inclusive exercise environment.

Once exercise groups are formed, exercise groups give moral support and promote accountability and encouragement. The community influences exercise by the safety level of the exercise environment and the number of opportunities for exercise, which includes sidewalks, green spaces,

playgrounds, and walking trails. Exercise provides several psychological benefits that can enhance overall well-being, including improved mood, better sleep quality, increased self-esteem, improved body image, and fewer depression and anxiety symptoms.

Behavioral Method of Training

Clients expect professionalism; building relationships and maintaining a facility that supports training competency is essential. Program designs should be tailored to the clients' abilities and address their health concerns and goals. Self-efficacy is one of the top factors that determine physical activity in adults; so trainers are required to focus on boosting a person's self-efficacy. Effective self-monitoring and planning are essential techniques in developing a self-regulatory strategy to improve self-efficacy.

Subjective patterns can impact a person's willingness to perform resistance training exercises. CPTs are expected to assess a client's stage of change and boost competency in fitness activities. The stages of change include reconsideration, contemplation, preparation, active decision, and regular activity. Both verbal and non-verbal forms of communication help cultivate professional relations between the client and trainer.

Listening actively requires a genuine interest in comprehending the client's health and fitness goals. A CPT has to ask appropriate questions, avoid distractions and inner dialogue, and provide the client with appropriate feedback. Motivational interviewing is a method of coaching that is used to enhance intrinsic motivation for change. CPTs sometimes use techniques from motivational interviewing, such as developing a discrepancy between a client's current and ideal state, initiating discussion about change, and assessing a client's willingness, and perceived ability to change.

A BCT aids in promoting the determining factors of human attitudes. CPTs may use numerous methods to enhance a client's confidence, motivation, or self-regulation skills through planning, goal setting and monitoring. Cognitive strategies that modify behaviors include positive self-talk, imagery, and the practice of psyching up before activity.

Goals set by clients ought to be **SMART. SMART** is an acronym for a **specific** goal, which is **measurable,** possible to **attainable, realistic,** and **timely.**

Process goals and outcome goals should be monitored by clients. For better results, clients should determine long-term bigger goals, then develop a series of smaller goals that promote the progress of the main goal.

Strategies to Strengthen Your Communication with Clients

Are you clicking with your clients? Effective communication is a two-way street, we all can improve a lot when it comes to our professional interactions with clients, especially new clients as we dance the often awkward dance of relationship building . Sharpen your rapport-building skills with the methods shared below.

Many personal trainers have perfected exercise and program design – they gather the necessary health and fitness information, create a plan, and then carry it out flawlessly. Unfortunately, we fitness professionals perform poorly in our abilities to develop rapport and proper communication channels with clients (Rapport Phase), and this becomes quite clear when watching PTs first meet prospective or new clients.

Building rapport is an initial and continual process, yet omitted by many trainers who direct their initial communication towards understanding an individual's needs and goals (i.e., gathering information) rather than making a connection. Not that this is irresponsible, but it is important to remember that rapport is instrumental to building successful professional relationships.

It is more than being polite and caring – it is the process of taking the time to actually show your care by developing a close and harmonious relationship. Eventually you'll understand their feelings and ideas, and can effectively and succinctly communicate to help them attain what they need and truly desire. It is a communion marked by harmony, conformity, accord, and affinity, and the overall relationship can stifle without it. However, it is also essential to observe that not everyone seeks or cares for rapport, at least not in the beginning. Here lies the true skill of being an excellent communicator. Effective communicators are skillful to recognize personality traits such as sociability, dominance) and ascertain how much communication is appropriate by adhering to the cardinal rule of treating others the way they want to be treated.

As fitness continues to migrate into wellness, every trainer of tomorrow will evolve to coach as well as training. Now, this will necessitate the acquisition of additional knowledge and skills, this boost in scope of service will undoubtedly increase the importance and value of fitness professionals. They will now be able to exert more influence in supporting and empowering individuals to meet their individual goals and sustain change. However, non-athletic training is very different and in NASM's recently-released [Behavioral Change Specialization (BCS)](#) these peculiarities, as well as the major responsibilities of coaches and trainers, are outlined. Some of these distinctive differences show how coaching is very reliant upon rapport, strong communication skills and empowering sustainable behavioral change.

Rapport relies profoundly upon effective communication, which consists of words, which simply relay factual information; and then voice tonality and non-verbal communication that pass the true emotion (meaning or purpose) behind the communicated message. Unlike the popular belief, where we were taught that words consist of only 7% of our communication in comparison to the tone and nonverbal communication that constitute the remaining 38% and 55%, respectively.

This is the 55-38-7 rule, conceived by Albert Mehrabian and colleagues at UCLA in 1967 to explain his research findings. He admitted that it was not intended to explain human conversation. However, as effective communicators, we need to attend to each and align each congruently so that we are seen as genuine, warm and trustworthy. It starts with us being honest, that first set of impressions we make about someone which determines the nature of the relationship moving forward. Michael Solomon and NYU Psychology professor, coined the '7-11 rule' where he estimated that people make 11 decisions about you within the first 7 seconds of meeting, and these decisions can forever shape the nature of the relationship. As professionals, successfully attending to five simple tasks can help shape those initial impressions to be positive:

• **Open** – your mental and body attitude. Do not be judgmental or adversarial. Open your mind - your reflex to give correct information will follow. Channel your heart towards the person to show that you truly care about him/her.

- **Eyes** – keep a relaxed gaze, because it puts people at ease. Spend 80-90% of the time looking at the triangle between the eyes and mouth. Looking away while having a conversation can be interpreted as submission or disinterest, depending on the culture.

- **Beam** – laughter and a genuine smile and are deeply rooted with making deeper bonds with people. They increase brain activity, releasing various compounds (e.g., endorphins, dopamine) that build more pleasurable experiences. But smiles must be genuine because fake ones are easily identifiable. A reak smile causes a slight eye wrinkle (action of the zygomatic muscles) and an upward lip turn – the reason for saying cheese. consistently try holding a pencil in your mouth between your lips (not teeth) to activate these muscles.

- **Say Hello** – your greeting and handshake gesture. Make your dialogue personal by using the person's name often – it also helps you remember them and other memorable stories about them. The handshake says a lot about someone; the firmness of the grip, the orientation of the hands, the use of one hand or both, willingness to shake, and more. When in doubt, slowly hold out a palm-open and upward-facing invitation and when the person responds, change your hand placement so that both hands are parallel to the ground.

- **Lean** – your body position should convey interest and connectivity. Lean a little bit towards the person but don't encroach into their space (18 – 48 inches distance is ideal in most traditions) and slightly imitate movements. If a person does not gesture as much as you do, this may prove to be distracting, just as it is if you're fidgeting or adjusting your body position while they are speaking.

Ask, Listen, Understand and Respond are four key skills to effective communication generally. It involves asking open-ended questions to learn about the person. It deals with active or immersed listening as opposed to passive or selective listening; understanding the true message being communicated by a person's body language and words; and lastly to respond only once you fully comprehend the situation.

To quote Steven Covey, author of the book *The 7 Habits of Highly Effective People*,

"Seek first to understand, then to be understood."

You should prioritise listening and understanding people during the rapport and investigation stages before we give any response. Many of us experience difficulty in differentiating between 'understand' from 'respond' and tend to listen with the sole aim of giving an answer (i.e., passive listening). But we should note that listening first can guide you to asking the million-dollar questions.

Listening is a form of art and our primary non-verbal communication skill. It captures a speaker's message and the emotions inspiring it. We humans are able to listen and process up to 500 words every minute in comparison to speaking about 125 – 250 words a minute; we are better suited to listening, and thus should do it more effectively. Various listening styles exist, each with their own individual characteristics, but active or immersed listening is what we should aim for as professional coaches.

Teaching yourself to truly listen is no easy feat. It involves practice and discipline. Put in the following strategies to be a better listener:

- Become more mindful – don't judge the message as it is spoken – don't get distracted by any emotional red buttons.

- Be attentive to all unspoken gestures and tone of voice.

- Control your external distractions – choose to meet clients in quiet places to cut down attention diversions.

- Tone down your internal chatter – tame the thoughts that distract you, such as thinking ahead about your answers or next questions. Inform the client and seek consent that momentary pauses will occur for you to take notes and form questions before you engage in any dialogue.

- Focus solely on the person speaking and avoid multitasking, for instance, writing and listening simultaneously. You will miss much of the unspoken message. Instead, use transitional pauses to make notes, reflect, paraphrase and think of your questions.

- Always ask open-ended questions that will help you gain more general information on the what, how, and why of a situation. More closed-ended questions are useful for summarizing or seeking specific details such as the who, would, which, will, and do.

A very effective skill set to use when communicating with clients is to find the connection between their current thinking and behaviors and how they communicate. In the NASM BCS course, the authors gave a unique angle on how to utilize Arnold Lazarus's Multimodal Screening (MMS) model as a tool for listening, the original intentions of developing MMS was to help practitioners understand an individual's thinking and behaviors (1). The MMS recognizes that humans behave (react/act), emote (have /express feelings), sense (respond to various stimuli), imagine (create sounds / images / events), think (beliefs / values / opinions / attitudes), and interact socially with others and termed these traits their BASIC ID:

- Affective

- Imagery

- Interpersonal

- Sensation

- Cognition

- Behavior

- Drugs (biological)

Two major factors for successful and sustainable behavior change are building the importance for change and its relevance to one's immediate life. When investigating, ask one simple open-ended question that will help you understand how their communication is linked to their behaviors or actions. Ensure to ask how their life would be different if they could affect the changes they desire and ask them to think carefully about their response for a bit. When talking with Peter, ask him, "Peter, with the challenges you have just shared with me, how do you suppose your life would differ if you managed to make these changes?"

For example, if Peter mentions that by losing 50 pounds he would be able to once again play with his grandchildren and it would possibly reduce the amount of back pain he has to bear daily, then he is connecting his communication to behaviors (playing with his grandchildren) and sensations (reduced pain). Whenever you need to make something relevant, or even find some additional motivation (when it appears to be reducing), use those same traits he expressed (i.e., behaviors, sensations).

There are many extra tools and strategies that effective communicators use to have good rapport with others. They are:

- Tone of voice – volume, inflection, speed, pitch, and rhythm. For example, when you end your speech on an upward inflection portrays doubt or a lack of confidence in what you just said, whereas ending on a downward inflection conveys authority and confidence. Try this example. Articulate the following statement out loud, using both upward and downward tones each time and note the differences in how you sound; "we will work on the project".

- Personality Indexing – it is a critical skill set needed to determine how to appropriately treat and dialogue with people. For example, individuals who score low on sociability tests do not value rapport initially or at any point in comparison with those that are highly sociable. With this knowledge, a professional can then attend to individuals accordingly (as they desire to be treated). Various indexes exist, including the DiSC Profiling, Myers-Briggs Type Indicator (MBTI), the OCEAN personality dimensions and Daves and Holland Model

A low socibility and low dominance person, for example, is more inclined to respect you more if you provide them with statistica and facts that appeal to their need to be correct and detail-orientated. Furthermore, they will really appreciate consistent follow-ups and a person who is well-prepared, detail-orientated and organized. Even how we communicate shows our personality styles – the rate at which we speak, and the conviction and frequency in vocal inflection gives insight into one's personality. For instance, a person who speaks at a higher tempo rate with higher inflections (i.e., energectic, animated, and charismatic) is probably highly dominant and sociable and values being stimulated by challenges, incentives, and rewards that are offered to them.

- Emotional Intelligence (EQ) – this portrays the ability to recognize and understand emotions, and how one uses this knowledge to manage oneself and relationships with others. EQ can be divided into personal competence and social competence. Each of these play an important role in how you sense and manage your own emotions in the moment while identifying the emotional states of others and managing those interactions successfully. It is estimated that the emotional quotient impacts 58 – 60% of job performance while the Intelligence Quotient (IQ) impacts a mere 10 – 25% of job performance. Roughly 90% of top performers in business possess high emotional quotient scores, while only 20% of the low performers have high EQ scores, illustrating just how important understanding EQ is to overall business success.

I should highlight a few of the major communication skills needed by personal trainers and coaches to thrive, and not barely survive as a professional. Even though many of us often believe we communicate effectively with others, we might be wrong. How often do we actually evaluate the true perception of our message by the receiver? Or the effects of our conversation?

As mentioned earlier on, effective communication is an art that can only be mastered with a significant investment of time, effort, and resources. Take the time to conduct a S.W.O.T analysis of your dialogues. Self-evaluate your Strengths and Weaknesses using evaluation techniques or feedback from others; identify Opportunities or areas for improvement, or showcase your communication skills; but never allow yourself to become complacent (Threats) by assuming you are an excellent communicator, or the message you think you are communicating is aligned with what you think your clients glean.

We often spend much of our educational resources and time focused upon the exercise sciences, yet we largely ignore what is probably the most influential determinant to our overall success – effective communication skills. It is high time we devise new training methods we train and retrain the way we think.

How to Help Your Clients to Stick to their Program

Jessica is a 42 years old woman who works 50 hours a week as a certified public accountant. She is also your newest fitness client. She desires to stop smoking, give up junk food and start exercising regularly—all the core essentials of a healthy lifestyle change.

6 months later, Jessica is still smoking and still lunching on pizzas. She misses workout days. Why can't she seem to exercise regularly or stick to a healthy eating plan? Jessica may not even know why herself. In such a case, then how can you help her change her habits? There's no shortage of health education campaigns admonishing her to change her ways.

They are not effective. What will work, however, is to help her use that education to make permanent habit changes.

Influencing Jessica's health behavior is much more important than creating exercise routines, making healthy meal choices, monitoring progress and being supportive. To help Jessica adopt and maintain a healthier lifestyle, you need to understand just how and why—and the theories behind behavior change science.

Understanding the Origin of Behavior Change

Where do you begin? Research encourages adopting a theoretical base for behavior change interventions because that will work better than a random, theory-free approach (St. Quinton 2017). When you incorporate the elements of a well-studied theory, you can identify the key factors and processes that affect people's ability to adopt physical activity and wellness strategies (Hagger & Chatzisarantis 2014).

A large amount of research has ventured deeply into behavior change to show why different interventions work for various types of people. Choosing the right theoretical base can be a vital step in developing successful lifestyle and fitness programming. But this is a huge task, owing to the overwhelming number of theories. This article will help you find some of the research on behavior change science and show you how to apply some of the most important theories.

The Four Paths of Behaviour Change

Up to 83 formal theories of behavior change have been developed, and more emerge all the time. That looks like a very significant number, but you don't need to know them all. The most extensively tested strategies are the Health Belief Model (HBM), Social Cognitive Theory (SCT), the

Theory of Planned Behavior (TPB) and the Transtheoretical Model (TTM).

• HEALTH BELIEF MODEL

The Health Belief Model focuses on how Jessica's attitudes and beliefs explain and predict her behaviors. The theory behind the HBM is that Jessica's desire to prevent illness and her belief that a specific action will help reach that goal will motivate her to take up healthy behavior changes. One challenge with the HB model is that people who do not usually feel susceptible to a disease are less likely to want to change their behaviors most times.

The HBM has been applied in the study and management of behavior change for 40 years, gathering a whole lot of empirical evidence of its success. A literature review found that up to 78% of studies exploring the HBM reported significant improvements in adherence.

The HBM has five core concepts, which are: perceived susceptibility, perceived benefits, perceived severity, perceived barriers, and cues to action . The strongest predictors of behavior are perceived barriers and perceived benefits. One of the biggest drawbacks of the HB Model is that it does not weigh the economic, environmental or socio-structural factors affecting change.

• SOCIAL COGNITIVE THEORY (SCT)

The SCT is based on a belief that behavior results from continuous interactions among environment, individual and behavior. It's built on the idea that when Jessica understands health risks and benefits, the power to change exists within her. If she, however, doesn't know how her lifestyle habits affect her health, then Jessica doesn't have much incentive to endure the challenges of giving up her unhealthy eating habits.

The Social Cognitive Theory proposes that behavior is a deliberate and conscious process for seeking positive outcomes and avoiding negative ones. It notes that while the environment can alter people's behavior, people can alter their environments to achieve desired outcomes. SCT identifies four major determinants of behavior: self-efficacy, outcome expectations, goals and socio-structural factors.

• PLANNED OR ORGANISED BEHAVIOR

Planned Behavior is one of the most well-researched and widely used theories that have been applied to exercise. Many literature reviews show its efficacy in predicting and explaining physical activity. The TPB combines clients' expectations about observing a behavior with the value that clients attach to that behavior.

The TPB defines four major psychological determinants that affect behavior change: intention (which deals with the client's willingness), attitude (it may be the positive or negative evaluation of performing a behavior), subjective norms (perceived social or cultural pressure), and perceived behavioral control. Of the determinants, the two strongest behavior predictors are intention and perceived behavioral control (perceived ease or difficulty).

One of the biggest disadvantages of this theory is the consistently imperfect link between intentions and actual behavior change. As Jessica's example shows, many people have good intentions but fail to carry them out.

• THE TRANSTHEORETICAL MODEL (TTM)

The TTM is a model based on empirical research results that shows people go through five stages of readiness before they change. To help Jessica work toward success, you first need to understand how and when she is likely to change her behavior. That will mean carving exercise programs to suit her current level.

How is that level noticed? The TTM recognizes five stages of the process: precontemplation, contemplation, preparation, action and maintenance. Progression through these stages happens in a cyclical, not linear pattern. Jessica may move to and fro depending on the stimuli and barriers she pertains to her situation. It's important to note that relapse is inevitable. And these unpleasant situations can teach Jessica how to stay in shape better.

For instance, you can explain that cyclical behavior is an expected occurrence and that she can always pick up where she left off. This novel and flexible approach, rather than the all-or-nothing view of behavior change is one of the biggest strengths of the TTM.

How to Choose the Best Technique

Just like each theory has its pros and cons because of its specific focus on constructs, stages, and phases, you would have to decide which focus is ideal for each client's nutrition habits they want to change unique goals, t, and so on.

The Health Belief Model, for instance, does not account for environmental and cultural determinants, while Social Cognitive Theory depends solely on regular interactions between people and their environments. So, if a client's lack of exercise is heavily influenced by his or her peers, work or family, SCT is a good technique.

Choose an approach based on the client's preferred outcomes and goals. First, identify the problem, the goal, and units of practice. Don't select a theory only because it is popular. A smart approach to selecting the right theory is to use a logic model of the problem, and with that work backward to identify possible solutions.

It is very vital for fitness professionals to stay within their scope of practice. Coaching has to do with a set of skills that are slightly related to, but separate from, those used in counseling, for consulting and therapy. Fitness professionals do not analyze a client's childhood, for example, but rather are focused on the present. Find methods of improving the client's current situation. And try to come up with solutions. The main target is for the client to "graduate" and continue in the established partnership.

Implementing Behavior Change Strategies

While behavior change is a conceptual foundation for exercise programs, behavior change techniques are the "active ingredients". The techniques represent the "smallest identifiable components that in themselves have the potential to change behavior.

The major behavior change techniques are premacking, contingency contracting, stimulus control, modeling, and relaxation training.

- **CONTINGENCY CONTRACTING**

It involves explicit agreements specifying expectations, plans and/or contingencies for the behavior(s) to be changed. This technique has four stages: set clear and precise target behaviors (like dietary activities and workout time frame and quantity), monitor progress, deliver consequences, and maximize generalization (establish reinforcing factors such as becoming a member of a healthy-eating group or getting a partner to exercise with).

- **PREMACKING**

This involves reemphasizing a desired behavior by pairing it with a likely behavior. For example, Jessica might organize a football-viewing party at home, where she could serve healthy snacks, instead of going to a sports bar that serves junk food and calorie-laden beer.

- **CONTROL OF STIMULUS**

According to evidence, we see that impulsive automatic factors drive many behaviors (Hagger & Chatzisarantis 2014). Thus controlling stimuli aims to reduce impulsive decisions. For instance, Jessica could carry along healthy food to work. This will help her avoid the temptation of going out for a pizza at lunch or grabbing free pastries during break time.

- **MODELING**

With modeling, Jessica would learn by seeing somebody else doing things she wants to do. Two forms of modeling can help people to change: behavioral coaching (that is, demonstrating and explaining proper execution of an exercise, having one's clients imitate it, and correcting their form) and learning to avoid peer pressure to eat foods that contradict the healthy eating plan).

- **RELAXATION TRAINING**

This type of training teaches clients tested techniques to help them find an ideal relaxed state. Examples are deep breathing, cued relaxation and progressive muscle relaxation.

How to Help Your Clients Overcome Behavioral Barriers

Being aware of the hindrances to physical exercise, right eating and other healthy habits is germane to helping clients change their habits for the long haul. Four primary categories of behavioral hindrances are:

- **Environmental**—space, climate and equipment

- **Social**—work, family commitments, lack of social support

- **Behavioral**—concerns about appearance, lack of interest

- **Physical**—chronic fatigue, generalized pain, body limitations

Note that clients often confront numerous barriers. For example, most life-threatening conditions in the U.S. are influenced by several risk factors, such as the consumption of alcohol and tobacco, lack of physical activity, and inadequate nutrition. Studies have shown that up to 92% of people who smoke have had at least one more risky behavior, and 9 out of 10 overweight women had at least two eating or activity risk behaviors.

Given Jessica's habits, you know she needs help dealing with multiple behaviors. As a result, basic nutrition guidance and workouts have to be "bundled" into one program. By this technique, can achieve more of her immediate goals (strength development, weight loss, etc.) while you cultivate the maintenance of these behaviors well into the future.

How frequently do we have clients stop their workouts after achieving their weight loss goals? That is the exact behavior we want to change. Putting into practice sound behavior change theories becomes central to making that happen. The behavior change science models examined in this article have been applied to healthy eating and physical activity with a degree of success. As a result, they can be applied to each one of your clients.

Do not allow your personal choices and familiarities dictate when picking a behavior change theory. Using a logic model can help your decision making. A good knowledge of a client's physical activities, eating patterns, and other healthy behaviors can help you prepare for the long term.

Client's goals are very important criteria for the behavior change techniques to be selected. A client might be more convenient and respond more to relaxation training, while another could prefer and work better with contingency contracting. You have to continually adjust your techniques as you monitor the growth of your client through the stages and barriers of behavior change.

So, yes, you can help Jessica succeed. With your new-found knowledge on the theoretical underpinnings of behavior change science, you will now be better equipped to aid your clients make a permanent change to healthy behaviors and stick with them for years and years to come.

Introduction to Cognitive Behavioral Therapy

Cognitive Behavioral Therapy is a sort of talk therapy that takes its roots from the idea that our thoughts have a vital role they play in our beliefs, behaviors and feelings. The goal of this sort of therapy is to change people's ability to respond to stressful and challenging situations and to change the way they feel, think and act. CBT brings to the awareness of your client their negative and inaccurate thinking, helping them have a clear view of tasking situations, This would help them respond more efficiently.

There are various types of treatments included in CBT, such as metacognitive therapy and mindfulness-based cognitive therapy. This has been applied in the treating mental health issues such as anxiety, eating disorders and depression. It has been used also to manage pain and stress.

Keep in mind that therapy is the profession of people with specific clinical training, professional experience and licensing. As a result, it is not something a fitness coach can do. Although you cannot conduct CBT with your clients, you can direct them to take guided self-help based on the basis of CBT.

Using the Multimodal Approach

Some people are better off employing more than one mode of behavior change. That's the principle advocated in the multimodal approach, which has been used in many areas, including life and health coaching.

Psychologist Arnold Lazarus created this approach in the 1970s. Rooted in social and cognitive theories, his theory holds that there is no system that provides a full understanding of human behavior or development.

The multimodal approach places focus on seven interactive dimensions, represented by the acronym BASIC I.D.: behavior, affect, sensations, images, cognition, interpersonal relationships, and drugs/biology. Many factors need to be factored in when applying this method: "What intervention, and by whom, is most effective for this particular person with that particular problem and under which set of circumstances?".

Using Motivational Interviewing & Positive Talks

Motivational interviewing is a form of collaborative counseling method that has seen a lot of success in obesity and diabetes interventions. Potency studies have shown that people who attend MI-based sessions in addition to complying with their regular interventions realized improvements in their adherence to physical activity.

With MI, the coach is a facilitator instead of an authoritative expert. The focus is on honoring and evoking the client's autonomy. It is vital to accept that the client is responsible for his or her own changes and cannot be coerced. MI contains four principles under the acronym RULE: Resist the righting reflex, understand the client's motivations, listen with empathy, and empower the client.

Thus, the coach shifts his focus on what clients can do rather than telling them to do something. Helping clients connect what they are passionate about with the motivation for growth can be helpful. For example, an older client may want to be able to play with his or her grandchildren and see them grow up.

Basic MI skills include asking open-ended questions, making affirmations, using reflections and summarizing.

This technique identifies how important the change is and the discrepancy between clients' current situation and where they want to be. Highlighting this discrepancy is at the core of motivating people to change.

STEP 1: USE "CHANGE TALK"

Sample questions: On a scale from zero to 10, how important is it for you to lose weight? Where would you be on this scale? Why are you at ____ and not zero? What would it take for you to go from ____ to (a higher number)?

STEP 2: BUILD CONFIDENCE IN THE ABILITY TO CHANGE

Sample questions: On a scale from zero to 10, how confident are you that you can increase the number of days you exercise? Where would you be on this scale? Why are you at ____ and not 10? What would it take for you to go from ____ to (a higher number)?

STEP 3: CHOOSE A CHANGE PLAN TOGETHER

Sample summary statement: It sounds like you don't want things to stay the same. We need to answer these questions:

- What do you want to do at this point?

- What changes were you thinking about making?

- What do you think you might do?

- Where do we go from here?

Using Technology to Enhance Changed Behavioral Patterns

Technology plays a critical role in changing behaviors. Posts on mobile apps and social media sites are also important accountability tools that keep clients on track and prevents the temptation to stray.

Social Media

Social media has become a lasting part of the public health landscape. The Internet has a lot of valuable resource for services that help customer's health ranging from online coaching for smoking cessations and weight loss to web-based appointment scheduling. While massive efforts seems to be directed at creating organizational tools for providing improved services for clients, peer-driven health communities have also been seen to be active on social media

There has been a long history of peer-to-peer interaction in the health sector, initially with the creation of support groups for tobacco and alcohol, weight control, abstention, long-term treatment, and grief and trauma counseling. The major advantage of peer counseling is the personal and empathetic interaction. The logic behind this sort of interaction has been moved into the virtual arena as online tools are developed for coaching and abstention. For example, web-based social support services such as Free and QuitNet and Clear give peer-to-peer e-mail and instant messaging systems that grant newly abstaining smokers counseling and support from people who have abstained for years.

On first look, it is an awesome development that anonymous online communities can be safe environments for providing meaningful interactions that aid the health behaviors of participants. The idea of social support isn't something new, even in the online space, it has been around since the start of the Internet since the 1990s; listservs and Usenet groups have used patient networks to provide tools for support groups to share medical information. For example, a long-standing Listserv for cancer patients and their families, ACOR, allows patients to share experiences through an open network to an empathetic community.

Radically novel approaches to social media as an instrument for improving health has gained popularity on social media sites like Twitter and Facebook.

For example, companies such as Healthways, Redbrick Health, and StayWell in order to promote compliance with planned health regimens, have begun to employ the use of social support platforms. These sites form communities that encourage increased participation in diet programs and exercise among their members through regular interactions and widespread recruitment. Recent Internet startup called PatientsLikeMe in the same vein offers a social media platform with patient information, online health profiles and disease histories, and interactive tools that create an opportunity for members to exchange whole report with each other.

Members of the website can participate in many disease-specific communities, giving them the chance to find information particular to their personal medical needs. Like Listservs and patient support chat groups from the previous generation, patients can exchange information relating to their treatments and experiences, but with the significant difference that the new, more refined social media technologies give room for participants to interact by comparing detailed records of treatment programs, ongoing health status, and recovery plans.

Added to the social support that participants receive, an important motivation for taking part in these environments is the novel informational channels that they foster across traditional health communities. A large amount of literature in social epidemiology studies the ways in which social, economic, spatial, and geographic constraints can significantly affect patients' health outcomes. This research has discovered that a major variable affecting population health can be knowledge about and access to medical treatments and technologies. For instance, studies have revealed that physician practices can be highly localized, varying dramatically from one geographic region to another.

Therefore, information about medicines, treatments, and screenings may be disproportionately available to some patient populations and not to others. The remarkable increase of Internet-based health and wellness communities provides patients with a variety of social and geographic backgrounds to exchange information about novel health resources, ranging from information about opportunities to learn about patient advocacy, diet and nutrition to , preventive health screenings, and new treatment technologies.

Through research, it has been discovered that social networking sites such as Instagram, Facebook, and health-specific platforms have been noted to affect the behaviors of people positively. Moreover, various studies looking into social networking and cognitive theory that those who engage the use of social media as a form of support for health-related changes, including increased physical activities and weight loss, had a higher success rate in behavioral change.

There are many pros fitness professionals can glean from social media sites.

First is the fact that these social media sites attract little or no cost. This enables it to be easily accessible to different kinds of clients on different budgets. It is also very flexible, it allows for the ability to customize programs to individual clients. This way, clients can get plans that perfectly suit them and their needs for the time. It is a great tool for ensuring that your clients stay up to speed with all the programs and exercises they ought to.

We also know that delivering behaviors change techniques over a plethora of modes increases their effect on health-related behaviors.

What's more, social media sites make use of clients' existing social networks, further pushing your clients to include behavior change into their daily lives.

Mobile Apps for Mobile and Healthiness

Health and wellness apps are mobile application programs that provide health-related services for tablet PCs, smartphones and other communication devices. There are several types of health and wellness apps that focus on multiple aspects of promoting digital health.

The most common categories of health and wellness apps include:

- Sports and fitness activity tracking
- Weight loss coaching
- Sleep cycle analysis
- Diet and Nutrition
- Pharmacy
- Medical advice and patient community
- Stress reduction and relaxation
- Meditation
- Menstrual period tracking
- Pregnancy
- Hospital selection and appointment management

The most common hindrances to exercise and healthy eating are lack of time and information. Many customers get overwhelmed by the task of preparing healthy food, tracking workouts, reading nutrition labels and monitoring calories. Fortunately, mobile apps have come up to help clients adapt.

Apps can be used to educate clients about diets and help in identifying healthy food choices when dining out. Apps can also keep track of food intake and exercise output and find places for seasonal produce.

Knowledge of these apps—and their usage—can aid you in showing clients how to overcome their obstacles to change. Another advantage of apps is their ability to keep you in touch with clients, remind them to take action, and aid them in finding communities that support them. Recent research shows that there is a rise in the numbers of people who are using online virtual health communities because they provide extremely important emotional support. And this is no surprise as the mobile health app market has seen steady growth in the past few years.

According to IQVIA, there are now over 318,000 health apps available in app stores worldwide. With over 200 health apps added each day, this is almost twice the number of apps available just two years back.

Health apps can basically be divided into three categories:

General health & wellness apps such as sleep apps that track our sleep patterns, nutrition-tracking apps that help us count calories, and stress-management apps that help us calm our mind, telemedicine apps that give virtual patient care by licensed doctors.

Health management apps that can:

1.) allow healthcare providers to share and report on a patient's personal health records remotely,

2.) assist individuals in monitoring their own health conditions, such as heart disease, diabetes, pregnancy, mental health, and more,

and

3.) help in keeping track of medications.

And what is similar amongst all of them? They help us live healthier lives!

A Reduction in Healthcare Costs

The gradual increase in the prevalence of chronic illnesses is costing the Canadian economy a lot of money yearly. Information from the Chronic Disease Prevention Alliance of Canada, the population of people living with at least one chronic illness is about 60% and those at the risk of developing one stands at about 80%. This comes at an enormous price to the economy.

Chronic illnesses costs Canadians $68 billion in direct healthcare costs. This sums up into an estimated $122 billion loss in indirect income and productivity for businesses. Simply put, preventable chronic illnesses are costing us and the healthcare system billions of dollars.

The good news?

Health apps are anticipated to reduce overall health costs for both providers and patients. The IQVIA Institute for Human Data Science carried out a study to assess the effect of consumer-focused health apps on the healthcare system in 2015 and concluded that "potential healthcare savings could be significant in the future". The study (focused on the U.S.) found that the usage of wearable devices and health apps could potentially save the U.S. healthcare system $7 billion per year.

This specific analysis focused on diabetes prevention, cardiac rehabilitation, diabetes care, asthma, and pulmonary rehabilitation, but it was discovered that if health apps were used across all diseases, that the healthcare system could potentially save $46 billion in annual cost.

That's significant.

Today, there are health apps developed to help control these and many more health conditions.

Why does this matter?

In the long run, this can diminish overall health costs for both providers and patients as an increased number of people are looking for preventative care to stay healthy.

Improved Efficiency and Speed of Healthcare Delivery

Health apps are making it easier than ever to manage, collect and monitor health information – from MyFitnessPal, a free app that allows people to monitor their calories and track their food intake, to Sugar Sense Diabetes, a free app that allows diabetics track their sugar levels, carbs, glucose, and more.

Similarly, patients who have heart disease can forward updated health information to their healthcare providers, and diabetics can track their blood sugar levels and relay the results to their doctor.

Personalized healthcare is now at our fingertips.

Ease of Data Collection for Health Care Providers

On the healthcare provider's side, these apps are also making it easier for professionals to collect and retrieve information from patients. Hospitals who use these apps allow these providers to access patient information, medical history, vitals, prescriptions, and lab results remotely.

Epic Systems, a healthcare software company, developed an app called PatientKeeper that provides physicians access to patient clinical data through either Apple or Android mobile devices. Here's a look at the app:

Instead of manually entering test results or filling out endless intake forms, apps like these can import test results and auto-populate the corresponding paperwork for health practitioners. They can also provide prescription advice and reminders, and help physicians avoid excessive testing and additional costs for patients.

Health apps make it easier for us to monitor our overall wellness as well as for doctors to treat their patients more effectively. Increasing

Convenience for Patients. This way, you can forget waiting in the waiting room.

Apps like a doctor-on-demand, Maple, Telemedicine app, grant us access to doctors anywhere, anytime. The modes of payment for services on numerous telemedicine apps are also quite convenient. Membership subscriptions to most telemedicine apps are either quite affordable or they are easily covered by a company's health plan

. Either way, a doctor you can reach out to at anytime is extremely convenient. From their homes, patients can now log into the app, get a diagnosis and treatment plan, and have prescriptions sent to their pharmacy to be delivered to them.

The advancement of mobile apps can have a great impact in reducing the spread of chronic illnesses, in turn saving the money spent on these illnesses.

Whether you are a healthcare professional or a patient, there are benefits to enjoy from health apps

Patients enjoy much more convenience with telemedicine than ever before. With features that allow us to monitor our nutrition, glucose levels, and a host of other health condition no matter the time of the day. With this advancement, we can now take the fight for our health a step further.

This new reality aids nutritionists; doctors, psychologists, pharmacists etc. improve their flow of work, and helps them to provide better services.

Overall, health apps are advantageous and promote a healthy lifestyle, and with time they would create more ways to improve the lives of many people in the future.

How to help your clients stick to their program through Goals Setting

You have probably been told these a million times. But what marks the difference between those who make headway and make positive changes and those who fail or are unable to make positive changes?

The secret is goal setting. Just confessing that you want to get fet does not mean much. How do you quantify being fit? Is there a standard for being fit? To truly aid your clients to succeess and truly make progress, you have to first inspire and motivate them by helping them to set the right goals; goals that can be tracked and measured.

Increase your knowledge base and better assist clients in making change. Make a difference that will outlive you! It is not always easy to achieve your fitness goals without a personal trainer. Sometimes you just lose motivation, and you can't seem to move forward. This is when you should begin to think about why hiring a personal trainer is a suitable option for you.

If you pick a personal trainer that has all the necessary qualities, you will start thriving again. There are various ways in which personal trainers aid you in fulfilling your fitness objectives.

What's more, even consulting a personal trainer online can be of great assistance, especially during times like this when staying fit at home is of extreme importance for your health.

What are the most common fitness goals?

There are various reasons as to why different people exercise. We have different bodies, our fitness goals are particular to us, and we all carry out our exercises in various ways. This is the reason many people decide to get a personal trainer to aid them in doing what they've set out to do.

However, as distinct as we all are, there are some fitness goals that surface quite often, that are similar or the same for many people. Let's see what those common fitness aims are:

- **Shedding fat** –The foremost most popular goal of many who decide to start exercising is their desire to lose fat. You should also get advice on how to adjust your eating habits, reducing carbs and reducing caloric intake, while you work out.
- **Building muscles** – While many people aim to lose weight, some want to build muscle so as to get a desired look and feel. To achieve this, they would need to increase their protein intake, go through long sessions of workouts, and involve themselves in plenty of lifts. Consultation with a personal fitness trainer is the best option if you intend to build muscles.
- **Improving Endurance** – A flight of stairs is enough to get some people breathing hard. To avoid getting winded easily, they start working out with the aim of improving their endurance. Having high-intensity exercises for 20-30 minutes intervals would be perfect for increasing you're your heart rate. You should work to keep your heart rate up.
- **Increasing flexibility** – A personal trainer should be your first point of call if your desire to exercise is to improve flexibility. They would be in the best position to assess your current state and how to move forward from there. However, you can still engage in some static stretches and PNF, but you should take note not to stretch through the pain and overdo it.
- **Toning** – Last but not least, some just desire to have a toned body. They are not in search of large muscles neither do they aim to shed so much fat. While this might seem easier than gaining muscle or shedding weight outright, it still requires a measure of discipline and a lot of effort.

Your workout clothes are very important. So no matter your body goal, make sure to be in clothing that does not restrict your movements.

The Importance of Setting Fitness Goals

Before you jump right into the process of goal setting goals and striving to get it, you have to comprehend the importance of what you are about to embark upon. This knowledge should not be alien to you as a trainer. Understanding the whys before starting a regimen helps you to achieve more result, this guides you to set the needed goals. This is better than going in without a plan.

To fully comprehend why goals are important and how they can help your client keep fit, you would need to explain to your client, help them see the advantages of getting a plan and exercising according to the set goals.

Goals Make Change Seem More achievable

For a lot of people starting a workout regime is a huge decision and one they had to summon a ton of courage to take. The overweight client in your office probably had to push herself to come for your training, There is the like hood that she has wanted to take this step for a long time now, but the task felt insurmountable for her.

To help her, encourage her with small, actionable goals, with this she will see that little by little change is a real possibility. It is not swimming the river, but swimming a couple of pools one after the other.

Goals Spur Motivation

A major challenge fitness trainer's face is keeping client motivated. Setting goals for your clients gives them something to hold on to, a next level to beat, and this helps them stay constantly motivated. Keep the goal, be it a specific weight loss or weight gain, or being able to complete a 5k without walking, dangling like a carrot and your client will be motivated for longer.

With Goals, You See Progress

This goes well with the idea behind motivation. When there are goals for your client to meet, you actually notice the progress you are making due to the effort you are putting in. If your clients goal is to get rid of a certain number of inches from their waist, for example, you can measure that. When they realize that the plans you have put in place coupled with their efforts are yielding results, this would act as a more motivation for them to continue.

Every Workout is More Efficient With Goals

Without a specific goal or goals or with vague goals such as losing weights or getting stronger, your client's focus during exercise sessions could be less concentrated than if there are specific goals such as losing specific amounts of weights or lifting a certain amount of weights.

With the appropriate goals, you'll help them save time by focusing on exactly what they intend to achieve and the strategies that will help them achieve this.

Without Having Fitness Goals, Success is Elusive

What all this points to is that success is more difficult to achieve when there no firm goals in place, You may shed some weight; you'll probably get a bit stronger; you will be much healthier than when you set out on your training; but will you achieve all you hoped for? Most likely not. To validate what you were hired for, your clients need goals to succeed.

Tips to Help Set Effective Fitness Goals

Having your goals set is one step, seeing your goals to fruition is a different ball game entirely. If you are searching for the easy way out, there isn't one. Having a personal trainer put you through the process is a huge plus, but you still have to put in the effort to see any change.

I want to swim faster; I want to be stronger; I want to slim down, these are not the ideal means of setting goals. As much as simplicity is good, too simple goals will not drive you to take consistent action. Good goal setting involves a lot of thoughtfulness. Proper time and attention must be given to the process of setting goals that will not end up in failure.

Take the resolutions made at the beginning of each year. It is a known fact that after the first few weeks of the year, the energy to stay consistent with the goals sets die. The truth is that many do not fail on these goals because they want to, rather it is because they are unable to properly set and stick to their goals.

1. Break your goals into parts.

A funny reason New Year's resolutions fail is because they are set too big. Aiming to shed 60 pounds by the end of the year is laudable, but it is not easy to try and achieve something so major. If you would really achieve that, you would have to split that goal into smaller chunks. For example, losing 5 pounds a month is a much more achievable goal.

2. Create goals specific and measurable

When you have clients with specific performance goals, they tend to do better. Why? They have very specific goals in mind. With specific goal, planning ahead is made easy and with specific plans, achieving your goals becomes easier.

Performance and Athletic goals can be measured. For example, on a race track running a certain number of miles within a given time. That is measurable, and you can focus training to achieve this.

3. Make realistic and attainable goals

Dreaming big when it comes to achieving your goals is not bad, but goals that are big and unreasonable would end in failure. If you are approached by a client who has very big goals, do not shut them down, rather help them divide the goals into smaller, more attainable goals.

Clients are more likely to give up when they realize their goals are unrealistic and frustrating to achieve. When their goals are broken down and they notice their progress, they are more likely to keep being motivated till they achieve their goal.

4. Put a time limit on it

A goal without a given timeline will not be achieved. When there are no time frames attached to goals, there is no sense of urgency around achieving them. If your client has a goal of losing eight pounds, when will they do this? The tendency for them not ever losing that weight is high. Set a bigger goal with a larger achievement time frame, like one year, and break this into smaller time periods.

5. Goals must be meaningful

The goals must have a personal significance and meaning to your client, if not, they have no desire to achieve them. You have to create an emotional connection, that is why it is encouraged to allow clients to set their goals themselves. You should provide guidance but never conclude on new clients by just assessing them without their consultation yet. Helping clients set goals is the first step in helping clients make lasting changes.

6. Set long-term goals

To produce results, you have to have a bigger picture first; a long-term goal helps you have a target. It could be getting a muscular body, losing fat, or improving your endurance. Have high goals, but do not make them too far from reality. You can trust your personal trainer in this process too.

7. Create short-term goals

With your long-term goals on the ground, you should create a plan to achieve them short-term goals broken up into monthly and weekly goals helps to motivate you and help you assess your progress better. Your fitness trainer can help in this regard too.

8. Measure your progress

Speaking of progress, find a way to keep track of it. While you can monitor your weight reduction on a scale, measuring your progress takes a little bit more than that. It involve you paying attention to achieving your short term goals and trying to avoid slacking off.

9. Make your short-term goals attainable

Coming back to being realistic – do not set goals that are too demanding to attain. You shouldn't let yourself take it too easy either, by setting yourself up for failure, you will only demotivate yourself, and you will hate the path you're on. A good Personal Trainer will help you to create the right goals.

10. Stick to the plan

Once you have drfted a routine for exercising with your personal trainer dont device from to it. It is vital to cultivate the habit of exercising out and to become responsible enough to carry out your weekly or monthly plans. Trainers help you stick to the plan.

11. Find motivation

Find a way to keep yourself focused through every goal, over every hurdle, and towards final success. Make sure you're doing this for yourself, not for anybody else, and be happy because of it. Your Personal Trainer knows how to keep you motivated.

12. Reward yourself

Finally, reward yourself for all the sweat you're putting in. Once you successfully complete a monthly goal, take yourself out. Everybody needs a cheat day once in a while and allowing yourself one after a month of discipline will only get you going stronger after it.

13. Understand what's driving your goal

Sometimes fitness goals are driven by insecurities, underlying fears, or body image issues—like desiring to run a marathon because you were bullied in middle school gym class, or joining a CrossFit class because an ex once commented on your size—and it's crucial to attend to these issues rather than thinking achieving your goal will appease them.

"Depending on what you are trying to accomplish, it can stir up a lot of emotions," says DiSalvo. It is advisable to visit a mental health professional if you get anxious when you think about your goal or if he thought of your goal triggers past mental struggles.

14. Be flexible in your definition of success

While you should have specific goals, it is also very important to keep in mind that those goals can be altered as you improve and grow into your fitness journey. It is quite possible a goal you thought to be very difficult initially turned out too easy or vice versa.

"If your definition of success is rigid, it will be hard to maintain that," says Vidal. Set goals you think you are achievable and then alter them as you find out more about your capabilities, Kollins Ezekh, certified personal trainer, group fitness expert and director of programming at Mayweather Boxing + Fitness, tells SELF. There's nothing wrong with moving the goalposts as you get more comfortable with your body's abilities.

15. Consider a professional's input

Finding it hard to place yourself on fitness level scale? Or is it difficult for you to form a realistic goal, and the process thoroughly overwhelms you, your personal trainer is the best person to reach out to, especially if he is certified. "A professional can help give you guidance on how realistic your goal is and can help you set markers along the way, so you can check-in and confirm you are on the right track over time," says Ezek.

At Fit Club NY, for instance, Scantlebury will ask clients about various factors influencing their lifestyle, including their prior history with fitness (e.g. Are they a former athlete? Have they trained before? Do they have experience lifting weights?), their nutrition, their work and social history (e.g. Do they go out frequently? Do they have a demanding, high-stress job?, etc.). These questions aren't to judge; they're to understand, explains Scantlebury. "Once we understand their life, we can create a program around that works for them."

On top of that, Scantlebury will conduct several athletic tests—like strength tests and endurance tests—to assess someone's baseline level of fitness. Though it is possible to pose this questions to yourself and take these fitness tests, if you're new to fitness, it would be helpful to get an expert's input.

16. Be honest about your prior and current habits

Asking yourself those tough questions can help you honestly evaluate what's most appropriate for you. Have you been somebody who in the past has crashed several fitness goals and just wants to take it to the next level? If that's the case, you could likely tackle a more complex goal, says DiSalvo, like running a long-distance race at a certain pace.

But if you're new to fitness, which of course is totally okay, you may want to focus on more simple behavior modifications, like going to the gym a certain number of days a week, says DiSalvo.

"If you want to see measurable progression, you have to be realistic with what you are currently doing," says Clancy. If your routine does not involve one form of exercise or the other, suddenly going to the gym five days a week—while certainly possible—might not be the most realistic or practical goal.

On top of that, taking a look at the past to identify what has stopped from previously achieving your goals is helpful. If you have a chronically hard time getting up in the morning, for instance, register for evening workout classes instead of aiming for those 6 a.m. sessions. Being truthful with yourself will help you pick out and eliminate barriers before you get started.

17. Plan for a support system.

When planning out your goal, you should also keep in mind those in your life who could motivate, encourage, and hold you accountable to it. Then let them know whenever you're in need of support. "If people you spend the most time with are supportive of your goals, it will make a huge difference," says Ezek.

Avoid These Common Mistakes When Setting Goals

Now you know that setting goals are not as easy s mny think. Goals cn be set in seconds by anyone but to do it correctly takes deep thinking and planning. Successful goal setting also needs avoiding some mistakes. Learn from mistakes others have made and stay away from these common mistakes:

Setting negative goals

Do not let your clients set goals like 'not being fat' or 'never eating junk food again.' Success is more attainable with positive goals like getting to a healthy weight or eating more vegetables.

Being afraid to adjust goals as needed

Adjustment doesn't mean failure. Ingrain this in your clients because failing is a big de-motivator. Always be prepared to change goals if you find they are not realistic or need more time.

Not tracking your progress

Record and document your client's goals and then have records of their progress over time. Do not forget that goals should be measurable. When you keep track of their progress, the benefits of their efforts become visible and this keeps motivation high.

Punishing failures

No matter the conditions, do not promote the concept of failure or attempt to punish your client. While this is usually a common reaction to unmet goals, this does not help your client. There is a tendency for us to punish ourselves when we don't meet our goals. Instead, speak with your clients on what could have gone wrong and how they can move forward efficiently from it.

Not rewarding achievements

While using punishments produces negative results, rewards can be rather helpful. When goals are met and when you notice progress from your clients, celebrate with them, it does not have to be something big, a simple high five might suffice in some cases.

Focusing on perfection

The concept of perfection is unattainable, thus focusing on it with your clients would dampen their spirits. Focus more on progress and consistency, not perfection.

Having fitness goals is of extreme importance if you want to make lasting, healthy changes. They should not be afterthoughts when dealing with your clients. When you meet a new client, you should steer your discussions in the direction of their goals. Do not take control of the conversation though let the client be in charge but try to guide and help shape their goals into more attainable, measurable, time-constrained, realistic and specific goals. Help your clients set up goals that will help them to succeed.

Practice Questions

How best can we describe instrumental support?

A. The support given by words of encouragement, empathy, and concern

B. The support that includes directions, advice, or suggestions given to clients about exercising

C. Individuals or groups that remove tangible barriers to exercise

D. The availability of family, friends, and coworkers to exercise with the client

Answer:

The Correct Answer is C. Individuals or groups that remove tangible barriers to exercise

The premise of instrumental support is to amplify the effectiveness and efficiency of intended outcomes. The best way to do this is by eliminating immediate barriers to success. While A, C, and D provide useful support resources, they are not instrumental.

2. What does the "S" in SMART goals stand for?

A. So precise the trainer understands its implication

B. Specific enough that any trainer could understand it

C. Specific enough that anyone can understand it

D. Specific enough that the client can remember it

Answer:

The Correct Answer is C. Specific enough that anyone can understand it

If a goal is specific enough for anyone to understand it even at a glance, it becomes easier to put into action. If the goal is understood by a trainer or trainers generally and it cannot be communicated with your client or laymen, it does not mean it's smart.

3. Which of these is an ideal short term goal?

A. Perform a hundred push-ups daily for six months

B. Lose weight to become a size 8 and wear old clothes

C. Lose 20 pounds to look good for a high school reunion

D. Research three reasons to exercise to support motivation

Answer:

The Correct Answer is D. Research three reasons to exercise to support motivation

A, B, and C are all goals that require habit formation and time making them long term if they are to be achieved realistically and healthily. A great short term goal can involve actual planning, which makes D the best choice.

4. What does "Realistic" mean in a SMART goal?

A. The client can and wants to work toward it

B. The trainer is confident that the client can reach the desired goal

C. This type of goal is completely novel to the client

D. It is a goal that the client is equipped to do

Answer:

The Correct Answer is A. The client can and wants to work toward it

B and C deal with a level of uncertainty that negates the realism being sought after. D is great, but the fact remains that a lot of people are capable of most things when it comes to improving their. It all boils down to willpower in that case. Therefore willingness and capability need to go hand-in-hand in order for a goal to be realistic.

5. How is the M in SMART goals effective?

A. Carving a time frame for the achievement of the goal

B. By making the goal not so tasking

C. By making the goal something they want to work toward

D. By making the goal quantifiable

Answer:

The Correct Answer is D. By making the goal quantifiable

The 'M' in SMART stands for "measurable", and from a scientific and even general perspective, the best way to measure a thing is through stats and numbers. This is what makes a goal quantifiable.

6. How does positive self talk aid the client's success?

A. It motivates the client to believe in their abilities

B. It compels the client to embrace exercise

C. It allows the client to succeed

D. It does not affect the client's success

Answer:

The Correct Answer is A. It improves the client to believe in their abilities

Positive self-talk is a powerful motivating agent. External motivators are great, but a person that can reinforce their own value internally would produce stronger internal motivation. C is the next best choice but is a very wide statement that does not give credence to the particular effects of positive self-talk.

7. Give one distinction between product and process goals?

A. Process goals give the client an aim to work to, product goals are goals to do for a point in time

B. Process goals can be predictively met, but product goals may or may not be attained

C. Process goals are achievable, product goals are often unattainable

D. Process goals are can only be attained with careful assessment, product goals are simple to achieve

Answer:

The Correct Answer is B. Process goals can be predictively met, product goals may or may not be attained

Process goals include behavioral shifts in mental attitude and changes. These goals can be anticipated based on evidence and feedback. Product goals are very specific milestones such as a specific body composition goal. The problem with product goals is the specific outcome may not be achieved, and due to the removal of the process adherence aspect, even once achieved, the client can soon regress.

8. Why should trainers ask for clients' permission before teaching them something?

A. Permission gives trainers freedom to share and speak their mind

B. Trainers must avoid sharing information with anyone unless they are permitted

C. It eliminates the know-it-all image from trainers and boost client-trainer relations

D. The client is paying for training and a thorough fitness training plan, not education

Answer:

The Correct Answer is C. It can eliminates the know-it-all image from trainers and boost client-trainer relations

The

quality of engagement in asking permission allows aliens to perceive the hierarchy dynamic between themselves and the trainer as more of an equal playing field. By requesting permission, you subconsciously ask the client to be a partner in the process rather than subordinate.

9. Which is not a behavior strategy?

A. Goal setting

B. Self-monitoring

C. Positive self-talk

D. Self-management

Answer:

The Correct Answer is C. Positive self-talk

A, B, and D are all behavior strategies based on habit-forming. Positive self-talk is not really considered as behavior as it is more of a tool towards motivation of correct behaviors such as the ones indicated in A, B, and D.

10. The most important thing a fitness goal should entail is:

A. The client should have a specific, desired outcome

B. Both trainer and client must believe in its feasibility

C. Both trainer and client should believe it is an essential goal

D. The trainer should design the goal, according to what benefits the client the most

Answer:

The Correct Answer is B. Both trainer and client must believe in its feasibility

Achieving a fitness goal is first and foremost a team effort, and that team contains the client and the trainer. While B and C are true, they are only correct when combined. D is incorrect because the client and trainer should both work on the goal. The client makes the goal and the trainer makes a plan towards it.

Chapter 8

Randomized Practice Questions & Answers

- Which sensory receptor does the body rely on when it is trying to regulate its temperature correctly?
- Nociceptors
- Thermoreceptors
- Mechanoreceptors
- Chemoreceptors

2. What is the main characteristic of motor (efferent) neurons?
- They are located within the spinal cord
- They process information from the dendrite and send it along to the axon
- They stimulate muscle contraction and create movement
- They rely on sensory receptors to recognize environmental stimuli

3. Of all the options, one of them is not one of the 3 major muscle types in the Human body. Which is it?
- Cardiac
- Skeletal
- Smooth
- Striated

4. Within the muscle, where does the exchange of oxygen and carbon dioxide take place?
- Within the capillaries
- Within the mitochondria
- Within the mechanoreceptors
- Within the myoglobin

5. If there is not enough oxygen when sprinting or when first beginning to exercise, which of the following is created?
- Pyruvate
- Acetyl-CoA
- Ketone bodies
- Lactic acid

6. Shoulder abduction is a result of the force-coupling between which muscles?
   - Pectoralis major and deltoid
   - Upper trapezius and rotator cuff
   - Deltoid and rotator cuff
   - Upper trapezius and serratus anterior

7. All of the following motions occur in the sagittal plane except:
   - Side bends
   - Triceps push-downs
   - Front lunges
   - Biceps curls

8. Which of the following initiates the electrical impulses that determine the heart rate?
   - Atrioventricular (AV) node
   - Atrioventricular bundle
   - Purkinje fibers
   - Sinoatrial (SA) node

9. Which of the following is not a characteristic of Type II (fast-twitch) muscle fibers?
   - Larger in size
   - Decreased oxygen delivery
   - Short-term contractions
   - Slow to fatigue

10. During a biceps curl, the triceps brachii would be considered what type of mover?
    - Agonist
    - Antagonist
    - Synergist
    - Stabilizer

11. Of the following options, which of them is not a characteristic of Type II (fast-twitch) muscle fibers?
    - Larger in size
    - Decreased oxygen delivery
    - Short-term contractions

- Slow to fatigue

12. In upper crossed syndrome, all of the following are overactive muscles in the head and neck except:
    - Levator scapulae
    - Upper trapezius
    - Sternocleidomastoid
    - Deep cervical flexors

13. What position does wearing shoes with a high heel put the ankle in?
    - A pronated position
    - A dorsiflexed position
    - A plantarflexed position
    - A supinated position

14. In what two ways should a fitness professional observe a client's posture and alignment patterns?
    - Statically and dynamically
    - Seated and standing
    - Supine and prone
    - Anteriorly and posteriorly

15. Of the following options, which of them is not a kinetic chain checkpoint term?
    - Knee
    - Foot
    - Core
    - Shoulders

16. Which of the following assessments would be most appropriate for an obese individual?
    - YMCA 3-minute step test
    - Rockport walk test
    - Single-leg squat assessment
    - 1-RM test

17. Which of the following is considered a best practice for a personal trainer?
    - Provide rehabilitation services for a client

- Prescribe a diet for a client
- Screen a client for exercise limitations
- Diagnose a medical condition for a client
-

18. Which movement-compensation might occur during an overhead squat assessment?
    - Knees moving outward
    - Head protruding forward
    - Shoulder elevation
    - Excessive forward lean

19. What might upper extremity exercise result in for an individual with lung disease?
    - Decreased muscular performance
    - Onset of dyspnea earlier than usual
    - Hypertrophied neck muscles
    - Muscle wasting

20. Of the following, which of them is not a cause of restrictive lung disease?
    - Asthma
    - Obesity
    - A neuromuscular disease
    - Fractured ribs

21. All of the following flexibility exercises are recommended for pregnant women except:
    - Active-isolated stretching
    - Self-myofascial release (SMR)
    - Dynamic stretching
    - Static stretching

22. Which of the following populations should avoid the Valsalva maneuver?
    - Individuals with hypertension
    - Youth populations
    - Individuals with osteoporosis
    - Individuals with diabetes

23. What is autogenic inhibition?

- A process where neural impulses recruit muscles for the production of force with the aid of the mechanoreceptors
- It is a process that involves the inhibitory action to muscle fibers leads to excessive increases in muscle length
- A process in which the tension impulses are much greater than the contraction impulses, that in turn leads to the relaxation of the muscle
- A process where proper muscle contraction is inhibited by excessive tightness of the muscle, leading to injury

24. Clients seeking strength gains should primarily exercise in what cardiorespiratory zone?
- Zone 3a
- Zone 3
- Zone 1
- Zone 2

25. Of the following, which of them is not a primary muscle of the global stabilization system?
- Quadratus lumborum
- Gluteus medius
- Latissimus dorsi
- Rectus abdominis

26. What makes "multiplanar single-leg box hop-down with stabilization" a balance-power exercise?
- It makes use of multiple planes of motion and requires full range of motion
- It requires stabilization in the jump from a platform down to the floor
- It requires dynamic control in the mid-range of the motion, with multiplanar movement
- It makes use of multiple planes of motion and requires force production followed by stabilization

27. What type of contraction do quick, powerful movements, such as those found during reactive training, involve first?
- Eccentric contraction
- Concentric contraction
- Active-isolated contraction

- Isometric contraction

28. According to the principle of adaptation, which of the following is true?
    - Adaptation allows constant improvements to occur
    - Adaptation requires a constant change of technique
    - Adaptation is represented as the primary goal of exercise programs
    - Adaptation involves the need for client education

29. When using the light-to-heavy system training protocol, about how many sets are in an exercise?
    - 10 to 12 sets
    - 4 to 6 sets
    - 1 to 2 sets
    - 5 to 8 sets

30. What is another term for the preparatory period in a traditional periodization model?
    - Proprioception
    - Intermuscular coordination
    - Neuromuscular adaptation
    - Anatomical adaptation

31. How many different core training movements should be used in each training session of Phase 1?
    - 1-4 core-stabilization movements
    - 1-2 core-power movements
    - 1-4 core-strength movements
    - 4-6 core-stabilization movements

32. What is the repetition range in the stabilization endurance phase of the Optimum Performance Training (OPT) model?
    - 15-25 repetitions
    - 8-12 repetitions
    - 12-15 repetitions
    - 12-20 repetitions

33. Which type of resistance exercises are specific to Phase 2?
    - Supersets with stabilization

- Supersets with power
- Resistance band movements
- Strength training with the barbell

34. What kind of flexibility work should be used in Phase 4?
    - SMR and static stretching with 1-3 sets of 1 repetition with 30-second hold
    - SMR as well as active flexibility with the 1-2 sets of 5-10 repetitions with 1-2 second holds
    - SMR and dynamic flexibility with 1-2 sets of 10-15 repetitions, with controlled tempo

35. Of the following, which of them is an example of a multi-joint exercise in the stabilization level?
    - Bench press
    - Standing overhead press
    - Two-arm medicine ball chest pass
    - Seated press machine

36. If an individual is performing self-myofascial release (SMR), what is the minimum amount of time to sustain pressure on a tender spot?
    - 30 seconds
    - 5 seconds
    - 10 seconds
    - 20 seconds

37. In pronation distortion syndrome, which of the following altered joint mechanics is present?
    - Increased knee adduction
    - Decreased foot pronation
    - Increased ankle dorsiflexion
    - Decreased knee internal rotation

38. Of the following, which of them is a concern during the ball crunch exercise?
    - Tucking the chin down toward the chest
    - Bracing the feet on the floor
    - Tilting the chin up toward the ceiling

- Allowing the back to extend over the ball

39. All of the following are acute variables for balance-stabilization training except:
    - Number of sets
    - Tempo
    - Rest frequency
    - Intensity

40. Reactive training enhances all of the following neuromuscular responses except:
    - Motor unit synchronization
    - Motor unit recruitment
    - Joint stability
    - Firing frequency

41. Which of the following best describes quickness?
    - The tendency to react with velocity to a stimulus and appropriately change the motion of the body
    - The ability to produce quick, powerful movements involving an eccentric contraction immediately followed by an explosive concentric contraction
    - The straight-ahead velocity of an individual
    - The ability to maintain a center of gravity over a changing base of support while changing direction at various speeds

42. Which of the following dictates the mechanical specificity of the training protocol for a client?
    - A client's fitness goals and physical capabilities
    - A client's metabolic function
    - A client's ability to use the appropriate energy system
    - A client's ability to recruit and synchronize motor units for firing

43. Of the following, which of them is an example of a closed-chain exercise?
    - Bench press
    - Push-up
    - Machine leg extension
    - Lat pull-down

44. Which of the following is an advantage of strength machines?
    - They improve athletic performance
    - Many of them move in one plane of motion
    - They challenge the core stabilization system
    - They offer multiple intensities in one weight stack

45. Of the following, which of them is an advantage of using free weights?
    - They provide extra support for special-needs clients
    - They require multiple dumbbells or barbells to change intensity
    - They permit the clients to move in multiple planes of motion
    - They may be less intimidating for some clients

46. Which of the following is the correct name of the training system in which an individual performs one set of each exercise?
    - Single-set system
    - Maximal-set system
    - Single working set
    - Single-exercise system

47. Balance is influenced by all of the following factors except:
    - Injury
    - Inactivity
    - Age
    - Weight

48. Which of the following is a total body stabilization exercise?
    - Squat, curl, to two-arm press
    - Lunge to two-arm dumbbell press
    - Ball squat, curl to press
    - Barbell clean

49. Which of the following best describes instrumental support?
    - The support expressed through encouragement, caring, empathy, and concern
    - They are the individuals or groups that take away the tangible barriers to exercise, such as transportation

- The availability of family, friends, and coworkers to exercise with the client
- The support that includes directions, advice, or suggestions given to clients about how to exercise

50. Why is it important to review previous exercise experience with clients?
    - It helps the trainer identify the client's weaknesses
    - It helps the trainer predict how successful the client will be
    - It assists the trainer in identifying the successful approaches to exercise
    - It helps the trainer identify poor form learned from previous training

51. How does exercise promote a positive mood?
    - Exercise brings out the best in people
    - Exercise can create happiness
    - Exercise creates positive thoughts
    - Exercise can trigger endorphin release

52. Which of the following is an example of emotional support?
    - Having a friend work out with the client
    - Complimenting a client for showing up and working hard
    - Giving the client feedback on their progress
    - Having a spotter at the gym

53. In which stage of the Stages of Change model would it be beneficial for a client to build a social support network?
    - Preparation
    - Contemplation
    - Maintenance
    - Action

54. If a client states that they want to win a step competition among their peer group, what type of goal is that?
    - Subjective goal
    - Process goal
    - Objective goal
    - Product goal

55. Which is the primary reason that certification is an important component of becoming a personal trainer?
- Having a certification can indicate the knowledge of proper assessment and instruction for safe and effective workouts
- It is important to most potential employers that a trainer has a certification
- A certification is required for reputability and is highly desired by potential clients
- A personal trainer is required to have a certification

56. Which of the following marketing P's refers to the communication information about a product or service?
- Place
- Price
- Promotion
- Product

57. Of the following, which of them is a major reason why a sale does not close?
- The trainer's personality did not mesh well with the client's
- The potential client was not seriously considering training
- The potential client was not able to express their goals
- The product or service didn't have enough value

58. Why is an accredited certification the ideal education option for an aspiring fitness professional?
- Accreditation is the pathway toward a degree in exercise science or physical education
- Third-party accreditation is the best way to ensure that the training is of good quality
- The certification with accreditation from a 3rd party is required by most gyms and health clubs
- Only the most experienced trainers have certification with accreditation from a third party

59. If emotions such as anxiety or depression become debilitating to a client, what should the fitness professional do?

- Direct such as client to a licensed psychologist or healthcare professional
- Call a friend or family member to alert them of what is going on
- Meet outside of their training sessions to provide social support
- Suggest the client keep a journal to track their feelings

60. Which of the following considerations applies to a fitness professional seeking employment at a large-scale commercial fitness club?
- Being responsible for their own client pipeline
- Having possible membership caps
- Having additional cross-functional responsibilities
- Focusing on sales

Answers

1. Which sensory receptor does the body rely on when it is trying to regulate its temperature correctly?
Answer: Thermoreceptors

2 What is the main characteristic of motor (efferent) neurons?
Answer: They stimulate muscle contraction and create movement

3. Of all the options, one of them is not one of the 3 major muscle types in the Human body. Which is it?
Answer: Striated

4. Within the muscle, where does the exchange of oxygen and carbon dioxide take place?
Answer: Within the capillaries

5. If there is not enough oxygen when sprinting or when first beginning to exercise, which of the following is created?
Answer: Lactic acid

6. Shoulder abduction is a result of the force-coupling between which muscles?
Answer: Deltoid and rotator cuff

7. All of the following motions occur in the sagittal plane except:
Answer: Side bends

8. Which of the following initiates the electrical impulses that determine the heart rate?
Answer: Sinoatrial (SA) node

9. Which of the following is not a characteristic of Type II (fast-twitch) muscle fibers?
Answer: Slow to fatigue

10. During a biceps curl, the triceps brachii would be considered what type of mover?
Answer: Antagonist

11. Of the following options, which of them is not a characteristic of Type II (fast-twitch) muscle fibers?
Answer: Slow to fatigue

12. In upper crossed syndrome, all of the following are overactive muscles in the head and neck except:
Answer: Deep cervical flexors

13. What position does wearing shoes with a high heel put the ankle in?
Answer: A plantarflexed position

14. In what two ways should a fitness professional observe a client's posture and alignment patterns?
Answer: Statically and dynamically

15. Of the following options, which of them is not a kinetic chain checkpoint term?
Answer: Core

16. Which of the following assessments would be most appropriate for an obese individual?
Answer: Rockport walk test

17. Which of the following is considered a best practice for a personal trainer?
Answer: Screen a client for exercise limitations

18. Which movement-compensation might occur during an overhead squat assessment?
Answer: Excessive forward lean

19. What might upper extremity exercise result in for an individual with lung disease?
Answer: Onset of dyspnea earlier than usual

20. Of the following, which of them is not a cause of restrictive lung disease?
Answer: Asthma

21. All of the following flexibility exercises are recommended for pregnant women except:
Answer: Dynamic stretching

22. Which of the following populations should avoid the Valsalva maneuver?
Answer: Individuals with hypertension

23. What is autogenic inhibition?
Answer: A process in which the tension impulses are much greater than the contraction impulses, that in turn leads to the relaxation of the muscle

24. Clients seeking strength gains should primarily exercise in what cardiorespiratory zone?
Answer: Zone 2

25. Of the following, which of them is not a primary muscle of the global stabilization system?
Answer: Latissimus dorsi

26. What makes "multiplanar single-leg box hop-down with stabilization" a balance-power exercise?
Answer: It utilizes multiple planes of motion and requires force production followed by stabilization

27. What type of contraction do quick, powerful movements, such as those found during reactive training, involve first?
Answer: Eccentric contraction

28. According to the principle of adaptation, which of the following is true?
Answer: Adaptation is represented as the primary goal of exercise programs

29. When using the light-to-heavy system training protocol, about how many sets are in an exercise?
Answer: 4 to 6 sets

30. What is another term for the preparatory period in a traditional periodization model?
Answer: Anatomic adaptation

31. How many different core training movements should be used in each training session of Phase 1?
Answer: 1-4 core-stabilization movements

32. What is the repetition range in the stabilization endurance phase of the Optimum Performance Training (OPT) model?
Answer: 12-20 repetitions

33. Which type of resistance exercises are specific to Phase 2?
Answer: Supersets with stabilization

34. What kind of flexibility work should be used in Phase 4?
Answer: SMR and active flexibility with 1-2 sets of 5-10 repetitions with 1-2 second holds

35. Of the following, which of them is an example of a multi-joint exercise in the stabilization level?
Answer: Standing overhead press

36. If an individual is performing self-myofascial release (SMR), what is the minimum amount of time to sustain pressure on a tender spot?
Answer: 30 seconds

37. In pronation distortion syndrome, which of the following altered joint mechanics is present?
Answer: Increased knee adduction

38. Of the following, which of them is a concern during the ball crunch exercise?
Answer: Tilting the chin up toward the ceiling

39. All of the following are acute variables for balance-stabilization training except:
Answer: Intensity

40. Reactive training enhances all of the following neuromuscular responses except:
Answer: Joint stability

41. Which of the following best describes quickness?
Answer: The ability to react with velocity to a stimulus and appropriately change the motion of the body

42. Which of the following dictates the mechanical specificity of the training protocol for a client?
Answer: A client's fitness goals and physical capabilities

43. Of the following, which of them is an example of a closed-chain exercise?
Answer: Push-up

44. Which of the following is an advantage of strength machines?
Answer: They provide various intensities in one weight stack

45. Of the following, which of them is an advantage of using free weights?
Answer: They allow clients to move in multiple planes of motion

46. Which of the following is the correct name of the training system in which an individual performs one set of each exercise?
Answer: Single-set system

47. Balance is influenced by all of the following factors except:
Answer: Weight

48. Of the following, which of them can be considered as a total body stabilization exercise?
Answer: Ball squat, curl to press

49. Which of the following best describes instrumental support?
Answer: Individuals or groups that remove tangible barriers to exercise, such as transportation

50. Why is it important to review previous exercise experience with clients?
Answer: It assists the trainer in identifying the successful approaches to exercise

51. How does exercise promote a positive mood?
Answer: Exercise can trigger endorphin release

52. Which of the following is an example of emotional support?
Answer: Complimenting a client for showing up and working hard

53. In which stage of the Stages of Change model would it be beneficial for a client to build a social support network?
Answer: Preparation

54. If a client states that they want to win a step competition among their peer group, what type of goal is that?
Answer: Product goal

55. Which is the primary reason that certification is an important component of becoming a personal trainer?
Answer: Having a certification can indicate the knowledge of proper exercise assessment as well as the instruction for safe and effective workouts

56. Which of the following marketing P's refers to the communication information about a product or service?
Answer: Promotion

57. Of the following, which of them is a major reason why a sale does not close?
Answer: The product or service didn't have enough value

58. Why is an accredited certification the ideal education option for an aspiring fitness professional?
Answer: The certification with accreditation from a 3rd party is required by most gyms and health clubs

59. If emotions such as anxiety or depression become debilitating to a client, what should the fitness professional do?
Answer: Direct such as client to a licensed psychologist or healthcare professional

60. Which of the following considerations applies to a fitness professional seeking employment at a large-scale commercial fitness club?
Answer: Focusing on sales

www.ingramcontent.com/pod-product-compliance
Lightning Source LLC
Chambersburg PA
CBHW081448070526
44586CB00019B/2270